WH
DOC

Dr Phil Whitaker is a practising GP and has been so for over thirty years. He is the author of several books and the winner of the John Llewellyn Rhys Prize, the Betty Trask Award and the RSL Encore Award. He is the medical editor of the *New Statesman*. He lives in Wiltshire.

@pwhitakerwriter | philwhitaker.co.uk

Also by Dr Phil Whitaker

Fiction

Eclipse of the Sun
Triangulation
The Face
Freak of Nature
Sister Sebastian's Library
You

Non-fiction

Chicken Unga Fever:
Stories From the Medical Frontline

WHAT IS A DOCTOR?

A GP's Prescription for the Future of the NHS

Dr Phil Whitaker

CANONGATE

This paperback edition published in 2024 by Canongate Books

First published in Great Britain in 2023
by Canongate Books Ltd,
14 High Street, Edinburgh EH1 1TE

canongate.co.uk

1

British Library Cataloguing-in-Publication Data
A catalogue record for this book is available on
request from the British Library

ISBN 978 1 83885 800 1

Typeset in Garamond Premier Pro by Palimpsest Book Production Ltd,
Falkirk, Stirlingshire

Printed and bound by CPI Group (UK) Ltd, Croydon CR0 4YY

FSC www.fsc.org MIX Paper | Supporting responsible forestry FSC® C171272

For Lucinda

And, of course, for Pippa and Robyn

CONTENTS

Introduction

WHAT WAS A DOCTOR?

1

MEDICAL RECORDS

I was seventeen and had not long passed my driving test. I helped my mum into the back of the car, her hands clutching a kitchen mixing bowl. It was the middle of the night; the south-east London suburbs were eerily quiet in the streetlamps' orange glow – this was 1983, years before the 24/7 society would begin bustling into eventual non-stop life. Occasional bumps or potholes caused Mum to take a sharp breath or let out a groan. I took every corner carefully but tried to keep up speed. Within twenty minutes I was turning onto the slip road, the headlights picking out the lettering on the large white sign: Queen Mary's Hospital. Next to that, the iconic blue NHS logo. I followed the red signage for A&E and parked outside the sliding glass doors.

The entrance lobby was brightly lit. The intensity of the glare seemed to make Mum's headache suddenly worsen; she winced and tried to shield her eyes. A nurse hurried over, took one look at her – waxen with pain and nausea – and ushered us along a corridor to an empty cubicle. The urgency of her response suddenly choked me. A few minutes later, the curtain swept aside. The casualty officer was over six feet tall, white-coated, with a folder in hand.

He glanced swiftly at Mum, his eyes appraising her, then laid a hand on her wrist to feel her pulse. I'd been running on adrenaline; my entire focus had been on getting her to hospital. Now, though, the doctor was here: calm, authoritative, efficient, purposeful. He looked over at me and suggested I return to the waiting room. The words conveyed something else: this was his domain, he would take it from here. The relief and the confidence he inspired made a profound impression on me.

So, too, did the candid glimpse I had of him an hour or so later, returning to his on-call room having attended to my mother. I was driving out of the hospital grounds, he was crossing the grass behind the A&E block. Those were the days of 100-hour working weeks for junior doctors. His gait was slow, his head slightly bowed. As he trudged, unaware of being observed, he shrugged off his white coat and slung it wearily over his shoulder. It stirred something my teenage self couldn't properly name. It lay in the juxtaposition – the capable, confident healer and the human cost behind the professional façade.

It was just a snapshot, I quickly passed him and was gone. I took with me from that night a sense of medicine as not merely a career but as a way of life. A vocation. A calling.

—

Dr Forshaw examined my wrists then propelled his wheeled chair back behind his desk. He tapped his pen like a drumstick against the wood. 'What have you done?' The question was posed under his breath; it was him speaking to himself. I couldn't even raise a wet flannel to wash my face anymore without excruciating stabs shooting up my forearms. It had been going on like this for weeks, ever since I returned from a post-A-levels cycle tour up through the Cotswolds to Stratford-on-Avon and ending in Bristol, where my sister was at university.

To see Dr Forshaw consciously working things out like that. The breadth of knowledge about the body that he must possess. He asked me to show him how I held my bike's drop handlebars. He emulated the position with his own hands. With a grunt of recognition, he reached for his green prescription pad. As he wrote, he tilted his head back slightly so he could focus through his half-moon glasses. 'Take these three times a day,' he said, tearing the top sheet off the pad. 'It's tendinitis. You've inflamed the tendons.'

He handed across the prescription. I hadn't planned to say anything but suddenly it seemed the right thing to do.

'I'm off to medical school soon.'

Dr Forshaw was the archetypal GP of the era – remote in manner, prescriptive in advice. He had been our family doctor from before I was born. On the occasions he would actually look at you, eye contact was brief and made over the top of those spectacles. He did exactly that then. He gave me a brief nod.

'You'll find lots to interest you.' He turned his attention back to his desk and started to write in my notes. 'It's a fascinating world.'

—

Caron, the practice manager, reached the landing and waited while I took the final few steps up the staff-only staircase.

'You'll be all right in here?' she asked, gesturing to an open doorway. The office was tiny, no more than a box room really, and dominated by a commercial-size photocopier standing against the far wall. But there was a single chair in front of a small square table.

'That's great, thanks.'

'Would you like a tea? Coffee?'

I smiled and moved past her into the photocopying room. 'No, thank you, I'll be fine.' I hung my jacket on the back of the chair.

'I'm just along the corridor,' Caron said. 'Let me know when you're done.'

I'd half-expected her to watch over me – medical records are important documents with legal standing and, while anyone can request copies, I've never heard of a patient being allowed to access their originals, not even if supervised. The fact that I'm a GP was perhaps sufficient reassurance, but if she'd had doubts then any of the partners in the practice – all of whom knew me well – would have vouched for me. Whatever the rationale for her trust, I was grateful to be left alone. I sat and picked up the Lloyd George envelope she'd put out on the table for me.

I've handled countless thousands of them over the course of my career. Made from manilla card, five by seven inches, the bottom and sides are ingeniously concertinaed so that the whole thing can be expanded to form a pocket an inch or so deep, allowing notes, correspondence, lab results and X-ray reports to be filed inside. They first came into use in 1911 as part of the 'panel' system founded by Liberal politician David Lloyd George – a health insurance scheme for low-paid working men. In 1948, when the Labour government under

Prime Minister Clement Attlee and Minister of Health Aneurin Bevan made the bold promise to provide cradle-to-grave healthcare, free at the point of use, for every man, woman and child in the country, those Lloyd George envelopes must have been the obvious design to adopt for the new National Health Service.

They're completely outdated. The subsequent explosion in modern medicine's ability to *do* things – investigations, screening programmes, surgical procedures, ever more sophisticated and complex drug treatments; our success in keeping people alive into very old age, often accruing multiple coexisting chronic diseases – has swollen the volume of material a typical patient will accumulate over the course of their lifetime beyond anything the designers of the Lloyd George envelope would have thought possible. When I entered general practice in the mid-1990s, receptionists had already become adept at splicing multiple folders together to create supersize notes to accommodate the burgeoning amount of documentation. That skill has now become redundant: computerisation means NHS general practice has become virtually paper-free over the past fifteen or so years, and medical records are now held electronically. Yet virtually all NHS patients still have a Lloyd George envelope (it was only in 2021 that newborn babies ceased to be issued with one). These iconic buff folders sit on carousels and shelves in every surgery in the land, untouched and undisturbed. If for any reason you want to go back in time, though, to see someone's medical history from before computerisation, you will need to get their paper records out of store.

The contents of my Lloyd George envelope were fairly

modest. Since my early teens I have been fortunate to enjoy good health. I delved into the folder and extracted the two treasury-tagged sheaves of paperwork from within. One was a collection of hospital correspondence – folded letters to and from consultants, pathology results, radiology reports. The other was a slim bundle of continuation cards bearing, in date order, the handwritten entries made about me by the GP who had looked after me as a child.

It was an eerie experience, reading my own medical records some four decades later, part of my quest to understand myself and what has happened to the profession I joined. There was the exact entry I remember Dr Forshaw making that day in 1984: 'FCU tendinitis. Rx diclofenac 50mg tds.' When I consult patients these days I put much more detail: a summary of the history, key examination findings, rationale for my diagnosis, other causes to consider if things don't work out as expected. I also note down important points from the patient's perspective: what impact the symptoms are having on their life, whether they have specific fears as to what might be going on. Then I map out the plan we've agreed together and what arrangements for follow-up or review we've made.

In part this level of detail is self-protective. In the case of a subsequent complaint or legal action – immeasurably more common than they were in Dr Forshaw's day – I would need my notes to evidence that I'd done a thorough job. They're also a communication tool. If a patient returns, I can swiftly remind myself of where we'd got to. And with the pressure to provide instant, convenient access, they might end up consulting with someone else were I not to be immediately available. In that case, I'd want a colleague to be able to get at least a sense of what had been going on rather than having to start the story from scratch all over again.

I leafed back through the continuation cards. There they were, almost all of them recorded in Dr Forshaw's fountain-pen script. I read them simultaneously as an experienced GP and against my fragmented childhood memories.

6 July 1976 (age 10). 'Labyrinthitis.' I remember him grasping my head and moving it rapidly this way and that, all the while peering at my eyes, looking for telltale abnormal jerking movements called nystagmus that would support the diagnosis as a way of explaining the dizziness I was experiencing. There weren't any. I could imagine how provisional the label would have felt to him. Vertigo caused by viral infection of the inner ear virtually never affects children. But he will have written it down as a 'best fit' – a way of describing what that episode of illness most closely resembled in case he needed to think about it again.

23 July 1976. '?appendicitis.' I recall him performing a rectal examination in an attempt to work out whether a 'grumbling appendix' could be the cause of the abdominal pain I kept being brought in with. The discharge summary from the subsequent admission was there in the other treasury-tagged bundle. The surgeon had convinced himself at the time of operation that my appendix appeared chronically inflamed. But that will have been wishful thinking. The path lab report filed in my records showed that, under the microscope, the appendix had proved entirely normal.

I must have posed Dr Forshaw considerable diagnostic difficulty, something I encounter every day in my own work. There were invariably serious organic diseases that could have accounted for my symptoms, and he will have been loath to miss something. I leafed back further.

1 May 1975. '? rheumatic fever' – a potentially serious complication of bacterial tonsillitis that can cause arthritis along with damage to heart valves. I was in hospital for days, traction weights attached to both ankles, until the doctors there were satisfied there was nothing untoward going on to explain my leg pains, abdominal pain and faint heart murmur.

Reading Dr Forshaw's notes, their brevity was a locked door: there was no way to tell what else might have been going on in his mind. Faced with the same situation myself – a child repeatedly presenting without biomedical explanations for their symptoms – I would be writing things like 'What's going on?' or 'Care here' to signal my disquiet and prompt deeper thought. I might draw in things I knew about other family members, who would generally also be my patients. But even though there was nothing in writing to prove it, I knew that for Dr Forshaw, with continuing care for me across the years, and with intimate knowledge of the family around me, each of those individual episodes must at some point have coalesced to form a story. When I looked more closely, I could see he had been back through the notes at some point and had numbered each of three episodes of apparent labyrinthitis I'd presented with over the course of fifteen months. He was drawing threads together.

It was Dr Forshaw who, in 1968, had diagnosed my father with testicular cancer. Dad was thirty-four and I was just twenty months old. Although nowadays survival is close to 100%, back then, even with the very best treatment, a third of men would be dead within five years. There were no ultrasound or CT scans; it was difficult to tell whether a tumour had already spread at time of diagnosis. Everyone was treated as though it had: surgery to remove the diseased testicle, and intensive radiotherapy to the lymph glands in the abdomen to try to kill off secondaries that might already have seeded. Dad underwent the same process. In hospital recovering from his operation, the patient in the bed next to him was dying, vomiting miserably, and with intractable bloody diarrhoea, the end stages of a cancer that it had not been possible to cure. A grim vision for Dad of what might be to come.

A junior civil servant, Dad had three children under five. He had a young wife who, as was the norm at the time, had given up secretarial work upon marriage in order to run the home and raise the family. Dad also realised, too late, that he had insufficient life insurance. With imminent death on the cards, no insurer on earth would increase his cover. Early death was frightening enough, magnified by the painful prospect of never seeing his children grow. And he was crippled by guilt about the financially bleak future his family would face should he be one of the unfortunate third who would succumb.

Not that I knew any of this as a kid. I remember him lying in his bedroom, tape recorder on. I could hear the disembodied voice of the therapist from behind the closed door, getting him to clench then relax muscle groups all over his body as part of relaxation exercises for anxiety. I found his medication bottle in the kitchen once, the label bearing the euphemistic term 'The Tablet'. Mental health problems were shrouded in stigma at that time. The name of the actual drug – probably an antidepressant like amitriptyline, or a tranquilliser like diazepam – will have been deemed too embarrassing to have been overtly on display.

Neither the drugs nor the taped exercises were sufficient. Dad was a volatile presence in the home – intolerant of the noisy chaos of three young children, unable to cope when even the slightest everyday thing went wrong. He would erupt with frustration or anger, shouting often, occasionally smashing something to give vent to the pressures roiling inside. Mum would usher us out of the way, entreating us to be quiet, telling us our father was unwell. I had no understanding, nor did I know that the tension that permeated the house was abnormal – it was all I'd ever known. Now, though, I understand what must have been going on. The minor symptoms any of us experience from time to time – a bit of diarrhoea, a twinge of pain – were invariably signs to him that his life was about to come to an end.

Dad lived with the constant fear that, any day, the cancer would return.

April 1975. My parents had closeted themselves in the front room of our pebble-dashed semi. It was where Dad had his bureau, in which he kept all his policies and paperwork, together with a lockable orange tin with multiple compartments, each topped by a coin slot cut into the lid, inside which he carefully distributed pots of cash to meet various categories of household expenditure. I don't remember doing so but I must have listened for a while outside the room before going in. It wouldn't have been possible for me to have grasped what was going on otherwise, not in the second it took them to stop talking when they realised the door was opening.

Dad was guiding Mum through all the financial information so she would know where to find everything after he'd died.

I don't remember how I reacted – the memories are partial and fragmented – but I must have been distraught. Mum, I think, tried to comfort me. Dad went straight out and returned a few minutes later with the brand-new bike they'd squirrelled in our neighbours' garage and intended giving me for my ninth birthday in a few weeks' time.

Another memory. Mum making me take a sleeping tablet after yet another evening repeatedly disturbed by me falling out of bed with strange dizziness. I don't think it was her medication; I think it was Dad's. I didn't want to take it, it scared me. Or, at least, Mum's terse, tether-end voice scared me. I pretended to swallow it but held it under my tongue. The pill dissolved and half my tongue went numb. That panicked me: I called repeatedly for her until eventually she returned. I told her what had happened. She told me to swallow the rest of the tablet down.

One more. Coming downstairs one night, treading ever so lightly on the stairs, going through to the dining room where Mum was sitting in a chair by the side of the gas fire crying like I had never heard anyone cry before. I don't know if I gave her a hug but I think I will have done. I must have asked what was wrong, because somehow she managed to get the words out: 'Sometimes I wish I'd never married your father.'

Dizziness. Tummy aches. Strange leg pains. I didn't make up my symptoms, not in any conscious sense. I was what would now be termed, by GPs like me, a child in difficulty. I was responding to the environment I was enmeshed in, an adult world full of insecurity, dread, emotional volatility, depression, withdrawal and pain.

—

Dad didn't die. Whatever symptoms he'd developed at that time must ultimately have proved to have been something harmless. I don't know how long it took for him to be given the all-clear – or whether he was able to believe it. By then he had seen his mother die of the disease, his father-in-law also. It must have seemed like cancer was all around. And it was not something people survived. It was not something even talked about in those days. People hardly dared utter the word, lest in doing so they invited fate to visit it upon them. To have been a cancer patient in 1970s Britain was to live emotionally isolated and somehow ashamed. How could Dad even have begun to communicate his feelings and fears when cancer was an unspeakable disease?

It might have been the sequential non-organic illnesses I kept experiencing, or perhaps it was my brother's intractable stutter, or maybe there was something else in our family's tableau. Most likely it was everything combined. The pieces slotted into place in Dr Forshaw's mind. I remember the stiflingly hot car journey, crawling along congested roads across South London: Bexleyheath, Eltham, Lewisham, Peckham, till eventually we arrived at the Maudsley Hospital in Denmark Hill. The therapist Dr Forshaw had referred us to got us children to draw pictures of our family. It was my sister who sketched the most telling illustration: three siblings huddled around Mum. Dad on the far side of the sheet of paper. On his own.

Mum still refers to it as his 'summer in the garden': the realisation of the impact he was having on the family completely broke him. He retreated outdoors, sometimes working the vegetable patch and fruit bushes, more often just sitting in a chair staring at *The Times* and only occasionally turning a page. Keeping himself out of harm's way. Eventually, at some point, he must have made up his mind. He came back indoors.

It might have been gaining popularity in America but in stiff-upper-lipped 1970s Britain – where men weren't supposed to have emotions, and certainly never to cry – therapy remained an alien concept and the idea of counselling had yet to be born. Dad took up the Maudsley's invitation to join a psychotherapy group, attending weekly sessions long term. I found a photo of the group a few years ago, mounted in one of my parents' albums. It was taken at a lunch to mark the end of the group's eighteen months together. Gathered round a table on the patio in someone's back garden. Four women, swirly patterned clothes, curly perms. Two men, Dad with his wide-collar shirt and Brylcreemed short back and sides. Incrementally, the demons that plagued him had been brought into the daylight and cut down to size.

This is no fairytale; there was no magical healing. Dad remained a traumatised man, and the spectre of dying a wasting death from metastatic cancer never really left him. But he understood himself better, and within the psychotherapy group he had experienced being understood by others. And with those things seemed to come more control. Life at home improved. The second half of my childhood was incomparably transformed.

—

What is a doctor?

When I entered medical school in 1985, I had role models that had given me a firm answer to that question. That nameless casualty officer was the doctor as heroic figure, there to render assistance in times of crisis, often at considerable personal cost. Dr Forshaw was the wise general practitioner, able to diagnose a huge range of conditions from minor musculoskeletal annoyances through to life-threatening cancers, and to take in complex emotional and psychological issues like family trauma along the way. The power of his practice came not just from knowledge and skill; continuity of care and a trust-based relationship were key. Over a period of years, you got to know and rely on your doctor, and your doctor got to know you and the circumstances of your life.

When I entered general practice in the mid-1990s, everything I encountered reinforced and refined what I believed about my role. I was not merely to be a next-generation Dr Forshaw, I was one of a new breed. Aloof paternalism was being supplanted by a new style of practice that sought to forge rapport and partnership between each individual patient and their physician. Holistic, patient-centred medicine was becoming the norm. At the same time, we were in the foothills of what continues to be a seemingly endless, exponential growth in medical advance. Never have doctors been able to do so much in so many diverse disease scenarios. The scientific education I'd been afforded meant I was well equipped to keep my knowledge, understanding and skills continually refreshed.

Yet now, as I enter my final decade as a GP, the answer to the question 'What is a doctor?' has never seemed more uncertain. Hospital practice has altered radically. The traditional 'firm' – tightly bound groups of junior doctors of varying degrees of experience looking after their particular consultant's patients – has vanished, replaced by teams who spin-pass patient care at every shift change. Consultants have become super-specialised, focusing on ever narrower areas within their field, with patients often finding themselves under multiple different specialists, none of whom is able to take an overarching view.

In general practice, continuity of care and trust-based relationships are in inexorable decline. Fewer and fewer doctors are entering partnership and taking on the long-term commitment to their patients that this entails. In many areas, practices have merged and grown to become impersonal mega-surgeries staffed principally by salaried GPs and locums who come and go. Patients complain of never being able to see the same doctor twice, of never knowing the person they're dealing with. Since 2015, successive governments have promised thousands more GPs to address chronic shortages, yet every new entrant is negated by a burned-out doctor reducing their hours or leaving the NHS. Gaining a consultation with someone, anyone, has for many patients become an almost impossible battle, with barriers and long waits the norm. New methods of access – online, telephone triage, 111, walk-in centres – seem to offer solutions, but simply serve to fragment care into disjointed episodes with the next available clinician.

No one seems any longer to hold responsibility for an individual's care.

This book is the story of what has happened to the role of doctor over the course of my career. There is no single story to tell. There is instead a multiplicity of stories, unfolding in parallel and interacting in unanticipated ways, each contributing to the reasons why my profession, and the experience of the patients it seeks to serve, is unrecognisable from when I joined with such idealism thirty-odd years ago. These different stories also illuminate what ails the NHS – a cherished British institution that appears increasingly unable to meet the nation's healthcare needs no matter how much we seem to spend.

We look back with incredulity on past eras of medical history, in which bloodletting, purging, mercury poisoning and mutilating surgery were undertaken with the best of intentions by our forebears. How will succeeding generations view our own practice? We are turning ever greater numbers of healthy people into patients. Potent pharmaceuticals are prescribed in ever more bewildering and often toxic combinations. Decisions over treatment are taken by professionals in disconnected silos, both constrained by and complacent about the guidelines that dictate what they should do. We have lost sight of the vital importance of relationship to medical practice, both to deliver cost-effective care and to ensure that humanity remains at the heart of what we do.

In diagnosing the causes of our current dis-ease, four imperatives emerge that will be vital if we are to free ourselves from the dysfunction in which we have become embroiled. These are challenges both for my profession and for those in government charged with providing the nation's healthcare. They will involve looking afresh at the encroachment of politics on medical practice, at the balance between specialism and generalism, how we manage the prevention of illness, and a fourth fundamental question that goes to the heart of our duty of care.

Central to these remedies are patients themselves. People whose voices continue to be drowned out by the din of political initiatives, organisational reforms, and commercial, academic and professional interests that have created our current crisis. With an understanding of what has happened to their healthcare, patients can demand that their voices be heard – in the consulting room, in their communities, and in the formation of policy by those who govern. These patients are all of us: you, me, your family, mine too. This book is for us all.

Part One

THE EMPEROR'S NEW CLOTHES

2

EDM

Simon's flat was the sort of place for which a visiting GP would need good directions. What had been described as a car park proved to be an irregular area of sloping tarmac enclosed by railings at the rear of a parade of shops that fronted onto the High Street. Vans for the florist and the bakery were parked next to each other. A cream-coloured Mini, its doors liveried in the logo of a local estate agent, was tucked in at the far end. Whether I was welcome to slot my car in alongside wasn't clear. In the end I reversed back out and left it on the road, in case the space were needed by some delivery vehicle that might appear while I was inside.

My shoes clanged on the treads of the steel staircase that zigzagged up the back of the building in the far corner. Were it not for the instructions I'd been given, I would never have thought of venturing up there. It felt like I was going the wrong way up an industrial fire escape. Which I was. But when I got to the top landing, things suddenly and surprisingly domesticated. There were pots and planters along the length of the metal walkway, filled with pansies and begonias and a couple of those foil wind-spinners you get at the beach. A bird feeder was suspended from a bracket around a gutter downpipe. And next to the aluminium-framed door, a painted wooden sign in the shape of a sunflower confirmed that I had found 24a High Street, and declared it to be Home Sweet Home.

Anne-Marie must have heard me on the stairs; she opened the door before I could knock.

'Thank you for coming.' She gave me a smile, but it didn't reach her eyes – worry and fatigue rather than unfriendliness. 'He's through here.'

She led me down a cramped corridor and into the living room. It was a big space, open-plan with the kitchen, but cluttered with equipment. My glance took in a Marshall amp, three guitars on stands and a synthesiser keyboard. Simon was lying on the sofa, still in his dressing gown, stubble on his face, his long greying hair gathered in a ponytail. There was an empty washing-up bowl on the floor and a faint smell of Dettol. The coffee table in front of him was littered with the familiar white boxes the hospital pharmacy uses for discharge medications.

I sat myself down on an ottoman on the other side of the low table. 'How are you getting on?'

He grimaced and laid a hand across his tummy: 'Not good.'

I started to gather details: when the stomach pains and nausea had started, whether he'd had anything like it before, if there were any associated symptoms like fever or diarrhoea. The range of possibilities was wide, anything from a nasty gastroenteritis through to a stomach ulcer, but as we talked, a pattern emerged. He was OK first thing but as the morning wore on he would feel progressively more poorly until, like now, he was fit for nothing more than lying there and enduring. It had been going on like this for several days. By the evening he would start to feel a bit better, so he kept thinking it would sort itself out, but it hadn't. He hadn't found anything that either eased or aggravated the symptoms. I quizzed him about mealtimes but no, he didn't think food made any difference either way.

'You've hardly eaten a thing since you got out,' Anne-Marie interjected, then looked at me. 'He's got to build his strength back up, hasn't he?'

I'd skimmed through his notes before heading out from the practice. The admission with chest pain. The urgent cardiac catheterisation – a long wire inserted through a vessel in the groin and threaded up to reach the heart – so that a stent could be used to reopen the coronary artery that had been blocked with clot. The cardiac arrest mid-procedure necessitating CPR and electric shocks to bring him back. How not all his oxygen-starved heart muscle had recovered even once blood flow had been restored by the stent. He'd been left with a weakened left ventricle, the chamber that pumps the circulation around the whole of the body bar the lungs. His ejection fraction – a measure of the heart's effectiveness – was little more than half what it ought to have been.

I checked him over physically. He looked pale, enfeebled, but beyond that there were no abnormalities to point to the cause of his symptoms. There was something else though, a sense of shellshock, vulnerability. A three-day hospital stay: heart attack, stent, sudden death, CPR, rib fractures, resurrection, home. I pictured him as he would have been just a couple of weeks before, mic on a stand in front of him, crashing out chords on his Stratocaster in the back room of one of the pubs his semi-professional rock band played at weekends. Now he had become a cardiac patient, acutely aware of his mortality.

I sat back on the ottoman. 'It'll be one of the tablets, I'm sure of it. Maybe more than one.' We both looked at the boxes strewn across the table. The drugs he'd been prescribed all featured in guidelines setting out how to optimise the function of his damaged heart, as well as to protect him from future harm. Everything had been thrown at him, no fewer than eight potent pharmaceuticals started en masse before discharge. I started sifting through. Aspirin could certainly be responsible: inflammation of the stomach lining is its most common side effect. But it's only a low dose required after a heart attack, plus Simon had been prescribed another drug to prevent it causing gastritis.

In any case, the pattern of symptoms didn't feel like it fitted. I sorted through the other boxes. Drugs to strengthen his weakened left ventricle. Others to prevent potentially fatal heart rhythm disturbances. Statins, of course. And still more tablets to protect the stents on which he now depended to ensure oxygen got through to his surviving heart muscle. Any of these could be causing the side effects. Yet, collectively, they represented a beguiling life raft, promising to keep him afloat. Which, if any, could safely be stopped? What alternatives might there be? Would they be as effective? If I started to unpick his medication regime, to dismantle that life raft, might I cause it suddenly to sink? And how might my cardiology colleagues react when hurriedly reviewing him in an overloaded out-patient clinic in a couple of months' time, when it became apparent he was no longer being managed according to protocol?

Just about to turn sixty, Simon should have years of life left ahead of him. He'd helped himself enormously by giving up smoking – 'I had my last one the day it happened,' he told me, and he sounded like he meant it. But equally important to the length and quality of the rest of his life was going to be this cocktail of drugs.

I glanced at Anne-Marie – Simon's shellshock made a second pair of ears indispensable – and agreed about the advisability of food, as much to cushion the impact of these multiple medications when they hit the stomach as anything else. 'But we've got some work to do.'

I set out a plan to change the times of day he took his tablets, varying one drug at a time. That way, if the side effects came on later, we would have tracked down the culprit.

'Once we've done that,' I said to them, 'we can see what we can do about it.'

—

Simon's story, set alongside that of another patient, Anne, who we'll meet later in the chapter, illustrates the impacts of a movement, evidence-based medicine (EBM), that has affected every aspect of medical practice over the course of my career. I was present at its birth in the UK and was enthused by its early, exhilarating promise. The fact that Simon survived his heart attack, and has a good outlook despite the damage done, is thanks in large part to EBM. Yet, as we shall see, its founding tenets have become hijacked and distorted, turning what was indubitably a force for good into the altogether more problematic creature we are wrestling with today – EDM, evidence-dictated medicine. To trace the origins of EDM, let us first turn the clock back to where it all began.

October 1985. The trunk was brand new, covered in burgundy leatherette with shiny brass fittings protecting its edges and corners from bashes and scrapes. I packed bulky and awkward items like my desk lamp and toasted sandwich maker in first, then filled the spaces with the rest of my gear, using clothes and bedding to cushion the Argos crockery and my motley collection of glasses and mugs. Fully laden, it was a two-person job to lift. My brother helped me load it in the back of his Austin Maxi, then we squeezed my bike, guitar and amp, and Z-bed mattress in around it. I glanced back as we pulled away. My parents were stood outside the front door, waving. Dad wore a neutral expression. Mum was both smiling and crying; I was the last of the brood to fly the nest.

The drive to Nottingham University, where I was to start studying medicine, took three and a half hours. At some point over the first fortnight I was taken, along with a bunch of fellow freshers, on a tour of the medical school library. The principal focus was for the librarian to introduce us to *Index Medicus*, the huge multi-volume bibliographic reference work, housed on rows of shelves along an entire wall, that we would need to become adept at using if we were to be able to search the worldwide medical literature for academic information. But my interest was also piqued by an exhibition room off the vestibule that we were briefly shown as the tour got underway. Once the induction into the mysteries of *Index Medicus* was over, I peeled away from the rest of the group and returned to look at leisure.

As a teenager, I'd been given a year's subscription to *Scientific American.* The article that most impressed me was a paper summarising all that was then known about different types of cholesterol and their roles in causing or protecting against atherosclerosis – the furring-up of arteries that results in ischaemic heart disease. I'd been fascinated by the intricate details that science was uncovering and the evolving understanding of the condition that was the leading cause of death in the Western world at that time.

One of the display cases in that Nottingham exhibition room housed a coloured plastic model of a coronary artery, de-roofed to reveal what was going on inside. What should have been a smooth tubular internal wall was roughened and distorted by a plaque, an inflamed area where mounds of 'bad' cholesterol had become deposited, creating a bulge into the vessel lumen, narrowing it and limiting the space in which blood could flow. This made sense from my *Scientific American* reading: this was why patients developed angina – chest pain when exercising. As the heart worked harder it needed more oxygen, but the furring up of the artery meant insufficient blood could get through. Angina pain ensued, and that made the person stop and rest. Oxygen requirements fell again and the attack resolved with no permanent damage having been done.

But that wasn't what the exhibition model was demonstrating. Where the plaque was bulging most acutely it had split the thin tissue lining the inside of the artery, exposing the inflamed cholesterol deposits beneath. Blood cells called platelets were shown beginning to clump and cover the rupture: the formation of a clot – thrombosis. The commentary described how, once that clot had started to form, it would swiftly and progressively expand until eventually it choked off all meaningful blood flow. The cardiac muscle downstream of the blockage would be permanently starved of oxygen and would die. This was different to angina. This was a heart attack.

The exhibit was accompanied by a poster describing a paradigm shift that was going on in the mid-1980s, one to which researchers at Nottingham had been making a significant contribution. For decades, the thing that had seemed most important to understand about heart disease was atherosclerosis, that process of plaque formation in coronary artery walls. But some researchers and doctors were beginning to think about heart attacks very differently, principally as a blood-clotting problem. This mattered because atherosclerosis, once formed, seemed an impossible problem to fix. But blood clotting . . . blood clotting should by rights be far easier to do something about.

What might have happened to someone like my patient Simon, presenting with a heart attack back in 1985, the year I started medical school? It would have depended critically on who his doctors were. Standard care would have been the same wherever he was admitted: morphine to relieve pain, nitrates to open arteries and improve blood flow, and potentially beta blockers to reduce heart rate and oxygen demand. But if 1985-Simon happened to come under the care of one of the minority of doctors beginning to be persuaded of the importance of thrombosis in heart attacks then he would also have been given immediate aspirin to thin the blood, and potentially an infusion by drip of another drug designed to further counter clotting.

Would that have helped him? No one actually knew. His

clot aficionado clinicians would certainly have believed so, but they were out of step with the majority of their professional colleagues. Conversely, might giving anti-clotting agents to heart attack patients actually make matters worse? Conceivably so: these are potent drugs that can cause haemorrhage. In the mid-1980s, how a heart attack was treated came down largely to a matter of belief on the part of each physician.

The only way to settle the question would be through scientific research, but that was a haphazard process. Papers suggesting that aspirin might provide protection had been appearing in the medical literature since the late 1950s. The initial reports originated from lone practitioners in America who thought they had noticed a strange but significant effect in their clinical practice – patients taking regular aspirin for rheumatic complaints appeared virtually immune to heart attack and stroke. These case series weren't well done in scientific terms, though, and they only found publication in backwater journals with tiny readerships.

The aspirin idea didn't go away, though, and over time it began to attract the attention of more academically able researchers who had a hunch there might be something to pursue. A definitive answer would require a randomised controlled trial (RCT) – pitting aspirin against an inert placebo in two otherwise comparable groups of heart-attack patients and seeing whether it made a difference to outcomes. But RCTs are expensive and aspirin had been off-patent since the Second World War, meaning it could be produced cheaply by any pharmaceutical company. No drugs firm had any incentive to fund research into potential new uses. A company that stumped up cash for an RCT would simply see its competitors gain should there be a positive result. University researchers did manage to win grant money to conduct small-scale trials, but their limited size meant they returned inconsistent results.

That state of affairs was overturned by the publication, in 1988, of a large-scale trial, ISIS-2, that had recruited some 17,000 heart-attack patients being treated in hundreds of hospitals internationally. The trial was organised by Oxford University, but funding to meet its huge expense came from Behringwerke, a German pharmaceutical company that manufactured a clot-dissolving drug called streptokinase. Like aspirin, use of streptokinase in acute heart attack had previously been investigated in several small studies, none of which had shown clear-cut benefit. ISIS-2 turned that on its head. Streptokinase turned out to reduce deaths from heart attack by 20%. And by astutely piggy-backing humble aspirin into the study, the Oxford researchers were able to show it also saved around 1 in 5 lives. Most excitingly, in patients who received both aspirin and streptokinase, the chance of dying from their heart attack was virtually halved.

ISIS-2 changed clinical practice. Before it came out, fewer than 1 in 20 UK coronary care units were treating heart attack patients with anti-clot drugs. A year after ISIS-2 was published, that figure had risen extraordinarily, more than two-thirds of hospitals now using aspirin and streptokinase. At that time, while I was still a medical student, such a rapid and widespread transformation in medical practice could only come about because of two interrelated phenomena. The clinical impact had to be dramatic in order to capture busy clinicians' attention: halving heart-attack deaths was certainly that. And the trial results had to have appeared somewhere they would be widely noticed. ISIS-2 was published in the *Lancet*, one of the UK's most prestigious medical journals. No one needed to scour the *Index Medicus* to find it; the *Lancet* is one of the few journals read weekly by a significant proportion of the profession. Doctors would come across the study and be impressed enough to alter their own clinical practice. And they would talk to their colleagues elsewhere – informally, socially, or professionally at meetings – helping to disseminate the new knowledge further.

It is just one example of the way scientific evidence advanced practice in that era. Across the whole slew of medicine – in fields as diverse as gastroenterology, surgery, rheumatology, neurology, oncology, psychiatry, general practice, public health – new treatments, understandings, approaches and concepts were constantly being tested and proven, devised and articulated. Each new insight had to jostle for attention, vying for space in the most prestigious journal that would agree to publish it. Proponents would take their work to conferences, presenting their findings direct to doctors in the same field from around the world. Drug companies with profits to be made would take out adverts in the medical press and ply the profession with information and free gifts, anything to make their novel product stick in practitioners' minds. And doctors had a professional duty, interest and pride in keeping themselves up-to-date. Most would seek out new information just as diligently as the thinkers, researchers and developers who were trying to attract their attention. The more impressive the impact on patient outcomes of a study, the more likely they were to alter their practice.

This was the way medicine progressed in that era: occasionally with spectacular leaps forward, more often incrementally and very slowly. Even the most incisive developments would take years to become standard practice. Looking back on my nineteen-year-old self, I could have had no idea how breathtakingly the pace, scope, methods and even ethical underpinnings of medical progress were set to change over the course of my career.

—

Simon came to see me after a second cardiology follow-up. 'He wants you to start me on this new tablet,' he told me. 'He said it would help with the breathlessness.'

I double-checked the letter from Dr Glenn, Simon's consultant, where he set out his recommendations.

'No, no,' I said. 'That's the one that caused you all the problems before.'

It hadn't proved easy to identify what was responsible for Simon's incapacitating stomach pains. We'd had a couple of false starts, first the statin and then the stent-protector drug appearing to be the culprit. Ultimately, though, they hadn't been. I'd begun to wonder whether what I'd thought must be medication side effects might in fact be manifestations of psychological distress. Simon's close encounter with death, and the way his life had been turned upside down, had left him anxious and low, sleeping poorly, appetite suppressed. Rather than trying to find out if there were a tablet to discontinue or change, I'd started to think I ought to be talking about how to help with depression. Then eplerenone, one of the pills intended to help his failing left ventricle, came into the frame. When I got him to stop taking it, the abdominal pain and nausea ceased. What's more, when I tried him with an alternative, the exact same problems recurred. He was intolerant of any medication in that class.

'Why would he have suggested going back on it, then?' Simon asked, sitting back in the chair and shaking his head.

I flicked back to Dr Glenn's previous letter from a couple of months before. There it was, written down in black and white: 'intolerant of eplerenone'. Yet at the very next clinic appointment, he'd recommended restarting the same drug. 'He must have got confused.'

I understood why Simon was peeved but I knew the realities. Dr Glenn's clinic will have been oversubscribed, urgent patients squeezed in, unforeseen problems with others already having taken up time he could ill afford to lose. Before calling Simon through he will have swiftly scanned the records to remind himself what problem Simon was there about. I could picture him going into 'heart-failure mode'. To begin with he'll have fired off questions about Simon's symptoms, gauging where on a standardised severity scale, the NYHA, Simon's case should be placed. NYHA classification is important in determining what treatments should subsequently be considered.

Then, while Simon was still talking, or had perhaps fallen silent, Dr Glenn will have been leafing through the notes to track down blood-test results, evaluating multiple features on Simon's latest ECG, checking how Simon's heart had been functioning on a recent scan. He will have been turning over multiple items of data, weighing them against guidelines – principally from NICE, the National Institute for Health and Care Excellence, but from other authoritative sources, too – and deciding what best to do. And there, in the drugs list in front of him, will have appeared an obvious explanation as to why Simon's breathing hadn't much improved.

He'd met Simon before, of course: once on a ward round in hospital, once at that first out-patient clinic appointment. But Simon was just one of hundreds of heart-failure patients under his wing. In the frenetic pace, with all the data he was assimilating and juggling in his mind, he'd overlooked that Simon couldn't stomach eplerenone.

Of course, the more Dr Glenn were to meet Simon, the more likely he would be to build a relationship and start to remember this kind of salient detail without having to scrutinise the notes. But next time Simon returned to clinic it was a different consultant he saw. I got a letter through: Dr Littlewood wondered if Simon might benefit from a different approach. As well as the plethora of drug treatments, pacemaker technology has evolved at pace. Sophisticated devices can now resynchronise contractions in the failing heart, improving its efficiency. Simon's ECG parameters didn't quite meet the guideline criteria for that, but there are also implantable defibrillators that can administer an electric shock in the event of a sudden rhythm disturbance, saving life. Dr Littlewood wondered if Simon might be eligible. He was sending him to Bristol for a cardiac MRI to help clarify.

More months passed, Simon returned to clinic after the MRI. Dr Littlewood offered him an implantable defibrillator.

'I told him: I'm not having it!' Simon came to see me afterwards, and sounded as though it had been an affront. I listened to his perspective. Whether it hadn't been explained, or he'd failed to grasp what are, after all, highly technical issues, he'd had no idea that the whole purpose of the cardiac MRI had been to assess his eligibility for an operative procedure. He'd assumed it was to give more information to guide his tablet treatment. But Dr Littlewood is a different breed of sub-specialist to Dr Glenn – an interventional cardiologist. His principal interest is in doing things with technology, rather than prescribing.

'If he'd told me what the MRI was about then I wouldn't have bothered to go.'

I checked he understood what the defibrillator might do: save his life in the event of a fatal rhythm disturbance. He nodded. Dr Littlewood hadn't been able to say how likely that might be to occur, only that there was some risk – though, equally, the medication Simon was taking already would provide some protection. It was unclear how much more an implantable device would offer in his individual circumstances.

Simon looked defeated, sitting there in the chair alongside my desk, his shoulders sagging. His previous abdominal symptoms had been due to medication, but I remembered starting to wonder at the time about other explanations.

'So there's no way you would go through with the procedure?'

The MRI detour might have been futile in terms of its original purpose, but it proved to be useful. Simon described the intrusive flashbacks to the experience in the catheter lab where he had died and been brought back to life. The mere mention of another invasive procedure on his heart had hugely amplified them: he was waking with nightmares most nights. It became apparent that he was suffering from a form of PTSD.

I changed the focus of the discussion. Were his breathing symptoms and fatigue more to do with psychology and less to do with his heart? Was a complete loss of confidence the biggest source of disability? He had panic attacks at the thought of going out; even coming to surgery had been a challenge. He'd yet to get back to the day job working for a family-run removals firm. Social life was non-existent. Anne-Marie was still in solid support, but things at home were getting frayed. And he hadn't so much as picked up a guitar in all the months since his heart had started to fail.

He readily accepted the idea of referral for psychological therapy. I was wary about additional medication in someone already taking such a lot of drugs – particularly when there was a small chance of them provoking heart rhythm disturbance themselves. But it would be months before he'd be able to access and gain any benefit from psychological treatment, so I felt duty bound to discuss antidepressants. I fully expected Simon to turn them down. As it was, he jumped at the idea.

Perhaps there was a boost from what we'd talked about – a relief at finally being able to express how he'd been feeling, not just how his breathing was. And maybe he'd known that there were things under the surface that weren't being addressed. Whatever the explanation, he paused at the door on his way out and gave a little laugh.

'You'll never guess what he said, Dr Littlewood, when I told him I wasn't interested in the defibrillator.' Simon smiled wryly. 'He only went and said I should go on that eplerenone thing again.'

—

It must have been one of his very first engagements. It was 1994, and David Sackett – tall, lean, with grey hair and beard – had only recently arrived in Oxford. I wondered what he thought of us, thirty young doctors ranged in front of him, all undertaking postgraduate training to become GPs – whether this was what he'd envisaged doing when he'd been headhunted from McMaster University in Canada. If he thought we were somewhat beneath him – Sackett was an internationally recognised physician and clinical epidemiologist – he never let on. He was charismatic and had no notes. For an hour he walked back and forth at the front of the seminar room, one hand in his pocket, the other periodically stroking his beard, enthusing about the movement he had been tasked with launching as head of the UK's first Centre for Evidence-Based Medicine.

Medicine had been striving to become more evidence-based for decades, with all the halting and contingent progress exemplified by aspirin in the treatment of heart attacks. When Sackett set up the CEBM in 1994 the World Wide Web was still a few years away, but computing power was already beginning to revolutionise the availability of up-to-date information. *Index Medicus*, that lumbering multi-volume beast filling a wall of shelves in my medical school library, had been turned into a searchable database as long ago as the 1960s, but now there was the prospect of it being readily accessible far beyond a limited number of users and librarians physically based at the National Library of Medicine in the US.

Sackett's arrival also coincided with the creation of the Cochrane Collaboration, a British-based but international movement establishing a new approach to evidence appraisal.

Panels of volunteer experts would examine the highest-quality studies about a particular topic in their field, arriving at authoritative statements called Cochrane Reviews, setting out what the literature demonstrated should be considered best practice for a given clinical scenario. No longer would an individual clinician have to identify and make sense of a range of evidence in journal papers, they could find a ready-made distillation from a group of leaders in that particular area of expertise.

Alongside these developments, personal computers were becoming more portable and powerful by the year. Many GP surgeries had begun to install them in consulting rooms and were starting to use them to systematise and improve clinical care. Sackett had spotted the potential for these different phenomena to transform the practice of medicine.

I still remember his original vision, articulated in that Oxford seminar room back in 1994. The doctor faced with a patient with symptoms of, say, heart failure, and asking themselves: what is the best thing to do to help? There would be no need to go to a library, a computer right there on the ward or in the consulting room would enable them swiftly to access the latest evidence. Often, this would have been digested and interpreted by leaders in that field. It would be like having the best minds in heart failure there by that individual doctor's side, helping to inform their decisions about the care of the particular patient, with all their specific characteristics, right there in front of them. Indubitably a good thing.

And in many respects, Sackett's EBM vision has come to pass. The descendants of *Index Medicus* can be accessed from a mobile phone, the latest medical literature hunted down anywhere. NICE now performs the role pioneered by the Cochrane Collaboration, convening panels of experts to appraise evidence and come up with recommendations. There is a NICE guideline covering virtually every significant aspect of medical practice, periodically updated in light of new research, setting out the gold standards of care. It doesn't matter where my present-day Simon might have been when he sustained his heart attack or developed his problematic heart failure. Any cardiologist in the land need only refer to the relevant NICE guideline (though in practice they will hold them in their heads) in order to know what the evidence says would be best to do for him. In that respect, David Sackett, who died in 2015, would be deeply satisfied.

—

Back at surgery, the lunchtime visits done, I set about working through the day's correspondence from the local hospital. Among the bundle, I came across a letter from a department called the fracture liaison service. They'd been checking up on patients who'd attended A&E over the preceding months with 'fragility fractures'. These are bones that have broken following only minor trauma – sometimes something as trivial as a jarring step off an unexpectedly high kerb.

My patient, Anne, they reminded me, had fractured her wrist following a simple trip. She ought to be taking medication to strengthen what must be weak bones. Only they'd discovered that she wasn't. They cited the relevant NICE guideline detailing what I should be doing for her and suggested I review her care. The implication was clear: I was failing to follow good practice.

They had a persuasive point. The next fracture could be something much more serious, a broken hip for example. Hip fractures are dangerous, with around 20% of patients dying within a year. They are also expensive: they require major surgery and rehabilitation. Among survivors, many never regain their previous level of independence and mobility, leading to increased care needs and costs long into the future. In not prescribing the recommended treatment to try to prevent such an occurrence, I was letting not only Anne but the wider health and social care system down.

I opened up her notes on the computer, not immediately able to put a face to the name and wondering how she had slipped through the net. As soon as I got her records up, the details came back. I could picture her in her pristine lounge: antimacassars on the chairs, silver-framed monochrome photograph of her husband, Philip, impeccably smart in his late-1950s national service RAF uniform, looking out at her from the hearth. She's in her eighties and has visits from carers four times a day, a situation that's been holding together for the past couple of years since Philip died. The wrist fracture had been manageable because her carers were already doing practically everything for her. But her domestic situation would never withstand a hip fracture. Assuming she survived, she would end up in a care home.

I clicked on the prescription section of her notes. The screen filled with the slew of medications she was already on. Multiple tablets intended to slow the progression of her mixed vascular and Alzheimer's dementia. Others to restore mobility robbed by Parkinson's. A hormone pill to ward off recurrence of the breast cancer she'd had excised the year before Philip had died. Then there were the laxatives to keep her bowels moving, and pills to control the distressing neuralgia she'd been bequeathed by a bout of shingles. These latter ones were by far the most important drugs to Anne personally, alongside the painkillers that lessened the daily discomfort from her widespread arthritis. Even these she had great difficulty remembering to take though, necessitating a dosing box, put together on a weekly basis by her pharmacy, that allowed her carers – who weren't permitted to administer drugs themselves – to prompt her to swallow the required medications at each care visit.

Should I prescribe yet more drugs, ones that would have to be taken at a separate time from Anne's other pills, and which could ulcerate her gullet if her carers weren't able to monitor her for half an hour afterwards to ensure she complied with very particular instructions? Or should I refer her for an intravenous infusion of an alternative product, with all the disruption and difficulty that a hospital visit would entail? She was eighty-two: a hip fracture was but one possibility among many of the next disaster that would inevitably befall her at some point. More likely it would be a stroke, or a fulminant pneumonia, or a recurrence of her breast cancer. By loading her up with more drugs, what would I be achieving? Would I be doing nothing more than tilting the odds between different causes of death for when her life reached its inevitable natural end? Anne lacked the capacity to take that kind of decision herself. But even before the encroachment of dementia, she had been the sort to look to doctors to advise on the best course. I had seen that with decisions about how best to manage her breast cancer. In the aftermath of her broken wrist, I had done the same regarding the question of bone-strengthening drugs: no way did I feel she needed yet more complexity and potential side effects. I decided not to prescribe.

Now, though, there was this letter. I looked at it again. It was medical shroud-waving. If you don't do this, it seemed to warn, your patient is bound to come to harm. And of course, Anne could quite easily catch a foot on a rucked-up rug one day, hit the ground and snap her hip just below the ball and socket. And there, filed away in her notes, would be this official letter citing the NICE guideline that, had I only acted on it, might have staved off exactly this catastrophe. Were anyone to look – a relative, a negligence lawyer, a coroner even – it would appear very bad.

No one ever sends me letters saying my patient is on too many drugs, though they could quite reasonably do so. The side-effect burden of many older, frailer patients' treatment regimes can be extensive and represents a great risk of causing harm. I had actually been trying to scale back Anne's prescriptions over the preceding two years. Gone were the long-standing blood pressure pills that had begun making her feel dizzy and faint when she stood, threatening falls. Her urinary incontinence was now being managed solely with pads, the tablet that had calmed her bladder overactivity potentially compounding her constipation and aggravating her dementia. And I'd jettisoned the statin she'd acquired following a brief hospital stay with a probable mini-stroke as pointless in the overall context of things.

But people do send me letters like this fracture liaison one. And NICE does keep churning out ever more guidelines that seem, with seductive certainty, to say what should be done across ever more health scenarios. The pressure is to do. Do this. Do that. Do the other.

Who might be upset if I didn't 'do' this latest thing for Anne? Not Anne herself, who would have viewed the complexities as being my job to work through. Her daughter, Mari, then – her only surviving close family member. I'd met with her several times and spoken to her on the phone many more. Whenever a problem cropped up – a new symptom, a possible side effect, uncontrolled pain, a treatment that no longer seemed to be working – Mari had to take time out from her professional and family life to be there for home visits or to accompany her mum to hospital appointments. She'd then liaise with the care company to ensure everyone was up to speed with whatever changes had been implemented, and that Anne's carers knew what to watch for to gauge success or failure. She was brilliant, Mari, but the task of coordinating her mother's care alongside everything else she had on her plate put huge strain on her and her own family.

Maybe I should contact Mari, arrange a phone call at least, talk her through the pros and cons and get her views as Anne's next of kin? That would, in many people's eyes, be best practice. But I felt in a quandary; I couldn't disentangle the conflicting strands. The pile of hospital post still to be processed was there in front of me. My afternoon surgery was soon to start. Everything seemed to demand a snap judgement: do or don't, prescribe or leave be. But it would have been just that, a snap judgement. I marked the letter to be returned to my tray after the admin team had scanned it onto Anne's notes. I would come to a decision at another point, when I had had more time to think. But even as I moved on with the day, I was aware of a lingering sense of unease.

—

Medical ward rounds as a student in the late 1980s followed a predictable pattern. The entourage would progress from bed to bed, the consultant taking presentations about each patient from junior doctors or students then agreeing or disagreeing with what they proposed should be done. There would be a woman recovering from pneumonia, a cirrhotic patient with decompensated liver failure, a chap with weight loss who looked like he might not have cancer as feared, but rather something called a connective tissue disease. A 1985 version of my patient, Simon, would have fitted right into the medical landscape of that era – someone with just one thing wrong with him, his heart. Someone with a single disease.

There, any similarities between then and now would begin inexorably to diverge. There were just a handful of treatments for heart failure back then, none capable of doing more than relieving symptoms. For the Simon of 1985, slowly and incrementally his left ventricle would have distended due to the backlog of blood it was unable to clear. Initially, stretching the muscular walls would have returned some of their power – picture an elastic band snapping back more briskly the greater the tension it is put under first. But there would have come a point when this situation failed, when the ventricle walls became so baggy they were less and less effectual – a vicious circle of decline. This process of 'remodelling' would eventually have caused heart failure so severe that Simon would have become breathless at rest and blown up with retained fluid. Death would have been near. In many cases, though, it wasn't the pump failure that would end life, it was a cardiac arrest – a sudden disturbance of heart rhythm, electrical signals gone haywire, so that it ceased to beat. Prognosis in heart failure when I started in medicine was so poor it was comparable to that for lung cancer: 95% of patients would be dead within five years.

Present-day Simon has an infinitely better prognosis, and that is down to the power of EBM. The decades of my career have seen ever better treatments. A few are old drugs which new evidence has shown to be valuable. Many are new products, the result of relentless pharmaceutical industry research and development, with well-conducted RCTs proving the benefit of each novel molecule. And implantable devices have brought new avenues with which to help, too. NICE evaluates all these interventions in great depth, stipulating which should be offered under what criteria.

Simon should live many years longer than his 1985 counterpart would have; his heart failure has gone from being a terminal illness to a chronic disease. Something that will very likely not much limit his life, something instead that he will learn to live alongside.

And as he does so, and grows older, he will develop other conditions. Perhaps prostate cancer. Then arthritis. COPD (chronic obstructive pulmonary disease) from the decades of smoking. Problems with his memory. Each has good treatments and need not be life-limiting, can be turned into yet more chronic disease. And each has its NICE guideline, its stipulations as to what to offer Simon. So as he moves into his seventies and beyond, he accretes more and more medication, more and more frailties and difficulties, becoming a patient, like Anne, who has suffered multiple assaults on their health and yet survived.

There were such patients – frail, complex, with multiple coexisting diseases – back in the 1980s when I trained. But they were few and very far between. Our ward rounds would come to them near the end, when we had been round all the patients with single diseases. The long-stay ward. A small collection of patients too frail and unwell to return home, but with multiple pathologies that medicine of the era could not improve. As I say, very few in that era. But harbingers of what was to come.

—

I picked up the receiver but paused before dialling Mari's number. I had a sudden premonition of what she was likely to ask me when I phoned to seek her views as to whether to prescribe bone protection to Anne. How much good would it actually do?

I realised I didn't know. It's the same with all guidelines: they stipulate what should be done but say nothing about expected levels of benefit. It can read like a certainty – do this thing and it will definitely work. But the reality is very different. The experts at NICE do have certain limits. They employ the notion of a QALY (quality-adjusted life year), an idea of what an intervention under consideration might achieve in improvement in both length and quality of life. If the cost is greater than about £30,000 per QALY then they won't approve funding – the reason we see periodic outcries about expensive new drugs not being made available.

But for Anne's bone-strengthening drugs the cost per QALY is minuscule so NICE is happy to endorse them. I called up Google on my desktop PC and used it to track down the source literature – doing exactly what David Sackett originally envisaged for EBM, only conducting the process in reverse. As ever when drilling down into original trials, results will vary. The very best-case scenario I could find was that the drugs being so strongly advocated for Anne had only a 1% chance of averting a hip fracture over many years of treatment.

The phone receiver was long since back in its cradle and I left it there. I could have phoned Mari, talked through the pros and cons with her, but how meaningful an exercise would that have been? I would just be passing on the same shroud-waving superstition that the letter had created in me. 'There's this drug that we could give your mum that has a 1% chance of stopping something really serious in the next few years, is more than likely to upset her apple cart in one way or another if we get her to take it, but: what do you want to do?' It would be nothing more than an exercise in self-absolution. Whatever happened to Anne would be down to Mari, not me. And if I struggle to weigh the merits and demerits of such dilemmas, how am I really to expect Mari to do better – especially with the emotional entanglements inevitable when dealing with your own loved ones and family. I would simply be abdicating the role I have decades of training and experience for, seeking to offload the dilemma on her.

As a young GP registrar in Oxford, I witnessed the inception of a movement. I wonder sometimes what David Sackett would say about the monstrous offspring EBM has sired. Guidelines and protocols – all based on evidence, certainly – gird every aspect of medical practice today. EBM has become EDM – evidence-dictated medicine. Fear of litigation, or even of simply appearing to provide substandard care, leads many doctors to view them as obligatory: things that must be done for any patient with that particular condition. Going against a guideline published by NICE feels like a risky thing to do. And as Simon's case illustrates, many areas of medicine have grown to become bewilderingly complex. Busy clinicians working under constant time constraints frequently focus on meeting the exigencies of the guidelines, never pausing to consider, along with their patient, what matters to them. The exercise of clinical judgement and the holistic focus on the individual are fast becoming dying arts.

Not only is guideline culture stifling the proper practice of medicine, it is also fuelling the epidemic of polypharmacy. The pharmaceutical industry has enormous financial muscle and it dominates the funding of clinical trials, which of course concentrate solely on studying the effects of drugs. As a consequence, the evidence base is hugely biased towards pharmaceutical treatments. The benefits to someone like Simon are substantial. But there is a significant downside. Pills are plied incessantly, and – as is so often the case now – when patients have several coexisting conditions, each with a different guideline dictating its management, the cocktails of potent medications can become huge, often to the patient's detriment.

In fairness to NICE, it has for some time been aware of the problematic culture it has helped to spawn. Some years ago, it appended this standard footnote to every guideline it produced:

> The recommendations in this guideline represent the view of NICE, arrived at after careful consideration of the evidence available. When exercising their judgement, professionals and practitioners are expected to take this guideline fully into account, alongside the individual

> needs, preferences and values of their patients or the people using their service. It is not mandatory to apply the recommendations, and the guideline does not override the responsibility to make decisions appropriate to the circumstances of the individual, in consultation with them and their families and carers or guardian.

It reads like a piece of small print on an insurance policy, and has achieved precisely nothing to reverse the widespread misapplication of guidelines as tramlines. Personally, I would prefer to see emblazoned across the top of every publication a far more provocative exhortation: 'If you find yourself following this guideline to the letter, you may not be doing your job properly.'

Even though David Sackett is no longer with us, I am confident he would be dismayed by the corruption of his EBM vision into EDM. Writing in the *British Medical Journal* in 1996, he explained:

> Evidence based medicine is not 'cookbook' medicine. Because it requires a bottom-up approach that integrates the best external evidence with individual clinical expertise and patients' choice, it cannot result in slavish, cookbook approaches to individual patient care . . . Any external guideline must be integrated with individual clinical expertise in deciding whether and how it matches the patient's clinical state, predicament, and preferences, and thus whether it should be applied. Clinicians who fear top-down cookbooks will find the advocates of evidence based medicine joining them at the barricades.

I'm sure were he alive today he would be leading the rebellion against EDM. And he would find delicious the irony of clinicians like me falling back on the founding principles of EBM to unpick the prescriptive assertions that now abound.

—

I didn't see much of Simon throughout the pandemic, though we followed things up periodically on the phone. The antidepressants were associated with a gradual improvement in both mood and symptoms, and the psychological work he eventually did – remotely via Zoom – was, I'm sure, even more fundamental.

His ejection fraction remains impaired, though the combination of drugs he's on has led to considerable gains. Quite what each respective intervention has contributed to the improvement in his fatigue and breathing and general wellbeing is unknowable and irrelevant – it's just good that it has finally come.

The band he was in dispersed during Covid, unable to rehearse or perform, and in any event he says he no longer has any interest in the lugging of equipment and the energetic performances it would demand. But following the reopening of pubs, he has played a few songs at open mic events. These days, he tells me, that is enough for him.

Anne never sustained a hip fracture. The impact of the pandemic on the provision of her care led to her being admitted to a nursing home. She died six weeks later, of causes unknown. Even in normal times a post-mortem wouldn't have been appropriate, and at the height of the first wave the Coroner's Officer was even more keen to agree a suitable entry for her death certificate based on likelihood from what was clinically known. I listed her various co-morbidities lower down the form and entered for the principal cause a description that is increasingly common: frailty of old age.

3

MÉNAGE À TROIS

Marta's HbA1c had come back raised for a second time.

'So what does that mean, exactly?' she asked.

Although this conversation had been on the cards for a while, now it was here I felt a momentary hesitation. As a blood test, HbA1c provides a measure of a person's average sugar levels over the preceding two to three months, but there are different ways of answering the question she'd asked. To begin with, I thought I'd better bite the bullet and explain the narrow medical interpretation.

'It means you've become diabetic.'

People vary in how they receive news like this. For someone who's been experiencing symptoms like inexplicable fatigue and has become worried about the possibility of cancer, a diagnosis of diabetes might prove a welcome relief. Marta, though, had not noticed any symptoms; her diabetes was 'silent', first suspected following an incidental finding on a urine test during a bout of cystitis. Others react more aversely: they may be apprehensive about needles and injections or have fears about suffering serious complications. Marta, however, appeared unperturbed.

'Well,' she said, shrugging, 'it is in the family.'

She folded her arms and tilted her head back slightly. She

wears large-framed glasses, through which she fixed me with a look.

I understood the defensiveness. There are genetic factors involved; her mum is a type 2 diabetic, which raised Marta's chances of developing it, though by no means condemned her to do so. While genes endow predisposition, most type 2 diabetes – the sort which generally comes on in adult life – occurs only once substantial excess pounds have piled on. The frequent link with being overweight or obese has been increasingly well aired in the media over recent years and with it has come the unhelpful insinuation: that this is a self-inflicted condition, indicative of gluttony and sloth, and patients have only themselves to blame. There can be a lot of stigma and shame. Launching straight into a discussion about Marta's weight – she was the best part of three stone heavier than she ought to be from a health perspective – was only going to backfire.

'You're right,' I said, 'it does tend to run in families. Tell me what else you know.'

Most of what she said was based on her mum, Matilde, who's also our patient. They're very close. Matilde moved to the UK when her daughter's marriage broke down. I don't know how long she originally intended to stay but seven years later she's still here, supporting Marta with her two boisterous boys and enabling her to keep working as a graphic designer. In return, Marta helps her mum with medical matters, accompanying her to appointments and occasionally, when Matilde's everyday English gets outstripped, translating more complex concepts into their native Portuguese. So Marta was braced to have to take tablets to control her condition, and she knew there would come a time when she might need to move on to insulin injections. She was aware that she'd have to come in regularly for blood tests, plus checks on her eyes and feet in case she was developing complications. Oh yes, and she would need to cut down on sugar in her diet.

I let her run through everything that came to mind. I wondered how much she felt actually applied to her. It can be an odd experience, being told by a doctor that there's something wrong – be that diabetes, or high blood pressure, or elevated cholesterol – when you feel perfectly well. And all that stuff about complications: nothing has yet befallen her mum, who's been diabetic for over fifteen years, other than some early changes in the backs of her eyes. Matilde is one of our many 'success stories': type 2 diabetic patients whose HbA1c levels we manage to keep in check. When she joined the practice she was already taking three different tablets, and her condition has followed a classic trajectory since. Her weight has gradually crept up, her sugar levels have become progressively more refractory, and she's needed several medication adjustments to keep them under control. Eventually, a year or so ago, other options having been exhausted, she went on to insulin injections. From Marta's experience of Matilde's condition, type 2 diabetes looks and behaves like an inexorable and incurable condition. Yet Marta seemed fatalistic. At some point while she was talking, she uncrossed her arms. She appeared comfortable on what was familiar and essentially unthreatening territory.

'You already know a lot about it,' I said. 'Tell me, though. Have you come across any stuff about diabetes being reversible? So you wouldn't need treatment at all?'

She frowned and shook her head. 'No. I haven't.'

She looked as though she was swiftly reappraising me. Marta has accompanied Matilde to any number of diabetes-related appointments. If there were some way of getting rid of the condition then didn't I think she would have heard about it? She does know me of old, though. Over the years we've had innumerable encounters – feverish kids, period problems, bouts of low mood. Just the humdrum stuff of life, but those repeated contacts have developed a relationship between us. Enough that she would give my words more weight than she might those of a total stranger she thought must be talking complete nonsense.

'Would you like me to show you?'

'Well, yes.' Her frown subsided. 'Of course.'

She shuffled her chair in closer to the side of my desk while I hastily sketched a diagram. I'm no artist. The stomach I drew looked more like an old boot, the pancreas an elongated sheep, and my graphical representation of a clump of fat cells inside the liver bore more than a passing resemblance to frogspawn. But it would do. I explained a simplified scheme for the two main types of diabetes. There is type 1, which usually comes on rapidly and at a young age, where the pancreas suffers permanent damage as a result of the immune system being induced to attack it, and it stops being able to produce any insulin at all. Then there is type 2 – her type – where generally speaking the pancreas is still capable of producing insulin, but fat deposited in the pancreas and liver interferes with its effectiveness, meaning it no longer controls blood sugar levels properly, something termed insulin resistance.

'You have to give insulin to people with type 1 because

they can no longer make their own. But your body still can, and if we get it working properly again then you'll no longer be diabetic.'

'And this is with tablets, yes?'

I shook my head. 'It's by getting rid of some of the fat cells that are causing the trouble – and it doesn't have to be all of them.' I struck a line through a couple of bits of frog-spawn. 'The way to do that is by getting your weight down. It doesn't have to be by much: five, ten kilos and you'll likely be cured.'

I put the pen down. She was still staring at the sketch. When she did look back at me it was with the same backwards tilt of her head, which was her way of bringing my face into sharp focus through her varifocals. She folded her arms again, an implacable barrier across her chest. Marta, it seemed, was set to become yet one more person with a chronic disease. She was on the verge of being swept up in the same evidence-dictated medicine (EDM) machine that we met in the previous chapter.

—

In 2012, Dr David Unwin was burned-out. He'd been a partner at his Southport practice for some twenty-five years, and the enthusiasm and satisfaction he'd once experienced as a doctor had largely evaporated. He felt disillusioned, stagnant, and the only thing keeping him going was the prospect of getting out – of taking early retirement in just a few short years, as soon as he turned fifty-five.

It was a consultation with an aggrieved patient that changed the course of his life. 'She came in and sat down and basically told me off,' he explained when I interviewed him for this book. 'She said: you've been prescribing me this metformin for years, and never once did you tell me I might be eating too much bread.'

Unwin's patient – we'll call her Joy – had joined the global diabetes community hosted by diabetes.co.uk and had come across a forum dedicated to a low-carbohydrate diet. Drawing on the experience of some of the 40,000 members worldwide, she had managed to bring her HbA1c down into the normal range and had kept it there even after she'd come off the drug she'd previously relied on for control.

'Hers was the very first drug-free remission of type 2 diabetes I had ever seen,' Unwin said. Chastened by Joy's ticking off, and curious as to how she had achieved the seemingly impossible, Unwin set about discovering more. He tried to join the same internet forum that had helped Joy reverse her diabetes but things didn't go well at first. 'I was investigated by the website's management and removed as a possible troll. In those days, most doctors were rubbishing patients' efforts to get well by giving up starchy carbs.'

Unwin's children found the idea of him being an internet troll 'hilarious', and during the investigation he evidently managed to convince the website's management likewise. It led to a friendship between Unwin and the online patient community that would in time have remarkable consequences. The more he learned about what people were achieving through adopting a low-carb diet, the more it threw his own practice into sharp relief. 'I realised I had lost my way. I was completely asleep, just simply prescribing.'

He sounded self-recriminatory when recounting this, but in truth he was no different to virtually every other doctor.

From my earliest days at medical school, no one ever suggested that type 2 diabetes might be reversible. When Matilde was diagnosed fifteen years ago, she will have been slotted straight into the time-honoured 'disease model'. Lip service will have been paid to dietary change, with recommendations to reduce sugar, sweets, chocolate, cakes and biscuits. But the height of anyone's expectation will have been that by curbing sugar intake it would make her condition a bit easier to control.

Instead, every action of the professionals caring for Matilde will have communicated a very different but unambiguous message: yours is a medical problem, it is up to us to deal with it. To do so we need you to take these pills, something so important that here in the UK, the government will exempt you from all prescription charges for any medication for the rest of your life. We will code you on our computer system to ensure you are recalled for frequent professional interventions: blood and urine tests and physical examinations to monitor your condition. As things worsen, which they almost certainly will, we will adjust and escalate your treatment accordingly. And when your pancreas finally burns out under the strain and is no longer capable of producing sufficient effective insulin, we will take over with injections. You are going to be a patient for the rest of your life.

This approach was scarcely questioned. After all, diabetes of any type can be a serious condition. It can cause illness – from minor symptoms like thirst, urinary frequency, fatigue, and blurred vision, through to vomiting, dehydration, coma and death. Even when patients are kept free of symptoms day to day, elevated sugar levels can, over a number of years, cause insidious damage to arteries, retinas, nerves and kidneys, the end result of which can be heart attacks, strokes, sight loss, amputations and renal failure.

With such a lot of hardcore health consequences, it's natural that doctors are involved. And in another of the landmark studies from the early days of the EBM movement, the UK Prospective Diabetes Study (UKPDS), there was apparently incontrovertible evidence that by keeping HbA1c levels tightly controlled with a variety of drug therapies, we could prevent some of the complications of the condition. Further evidence accrued that by prescribing additional medication to reduce high blood pressure, and statins to ward off atherosclerosis – both of which frequently develop in the context of diabetes – we could protect kidney function and further reduce the risk of heart attacks and strokes. Everything in the medical literature reinforced the sense that type 2 diabetes is most assuredly a medical problem, and EBM kept adding to the panoply of therapies we should use to counter its effects.

David Unwin's encounters with the low-carb community inspired a very different understanding. Those people genetically susceptible to type 2 diabetes (and there are a lot) simply cannot handle the amount of sugar being taken into their bodies. Their diet is poisoning them. The more deeply Unwin delved into the topic, the more perturbed he became. 'I asked myself: where does all the sugar come from?' The obvious candidates – the spoonfuls of white crystals dissolved in beverages or scattered over breakfast cereals, the sweets and chocolate bars arrayed in front of shoppers as they approach the tills – were but the tip of the iceberg. There are large quantities of sugar 'hidden' in processed foods and drinks. And most surprising of all, apparently neutral foods such as rice, pasta and bread turned out to resemble Trojan horses. 'The starch they contain is comprised of glucose molecules "holding hands" in long chains.' They don't taste sweet when we eat them, but once digestion gets underway, they release a surge of sugar directly into the blood stream. 'I became obsessed with the GI index and glycaemic load,' Unwin said, referring to measures that reflect the amount of sugar different foodstuffs contain and the rapidity with which it is absorbed from the gut.

There was something else that helped spur Unwin into action. In 1986 – when I was at the beginning of my medical training, and shortly after he became a GP partner – Unwin's Southport surgery had conducted an audit of their type 2 diabetic patients. 'There were fifty-seven of them in a practice of nine thousand,' he recalled, 'all of whom were over the age of fifty-five.' When he repeated the exercise twenty-five years later, he found a dramatically different picture. Despite the list size being virtually the same, the surgery now had well over 400 type 2 diabetics. The eight-fold increase was startling enough, but so too was the changing demographic: the new wave of type 2 diabetics was noticeably younger, many under the age of thirty-five. Given that complications develop over a period of years, the longer someone lives with the condition, the more chance they have of coming to grief.

Unwin's practice was entirely typical. My own surgery saw a comparable eightfold rise in the numbers of patients with type 2 diabetes over the same timeframe, and nationally Diabetes UK estimates approximately 4.5 million of us now have the condition. In our area, at the same time that Unwin was evolving his new understanding, we were having crisis meetings convened by our local diabetes consultants. The hospital clinics, where we would send the most complex patients, were overwhelmed and could no longer cope with the demand. They proposed new service models to support GPs in managing even the most challenging of these cases without referral, instituting a programme of outreach visits by consultants to guide difficult decisions over medication adjustments as people's sugar levels became ever more resistant to treatment over time. We were – GPs and consultants alike – firmly stuck in our disease-model thinking and paralysed by the sheer scale of the epidemic engulfing us. In Southport, though, Unwin was about to embark on a radically different course. It was one that would see him meet huge resistance and even vilification. But as he put it: when he sat looking at the stark results of his re-audit it struck him that 'something dreadful had occurred. And I realised drugs were unlikely to be the answer'.

—

Marta left the consultation on good terms. I respected her tacit instruction that her weight was not currently up for discussion. In return, she resolved to cut back on sugary snacks and Fanta. We agreed a repeat HbA1c in three months' time to see where she'd managed to get to. Experience told me it wouldn't be enough, that we were going to be starting medication sometime soon. But I didn't want to just then. I'd not given up on trying to avoid the disease model.

As she got up to go, I asked if she would like to take my 'basics of diabetes' diagram with her, which she graciously accepted. I said I didn't think it would fetch much on the art market. That made her laugh and she got me to sign it. I didn't know whether she would keep it or not, maybe she would stick it in a drawer and only rediscover it years hence when she came to move home. But in giving her my scrappy drawing, I hoped the visual image might remain in the back of her mind and encourage or motivate her to think further on what we'd talked about.

After she'd gone, I turned to my computer and added the code for type 2 diabetes to her records. To a casual observer, it would have looked like I was doing what doctors have been doing for centuries: diagnosing a disease. But that would be too simplistic. What I was actually doing – just like countless colleagues up and down the country every day, whether aware of it or not – was something far more complicated and double-edged.

The presence of that computer code added Marta to our practice diabetes register. This is a good thing. It allows us to identify all our type 2 patients. We can then audit the standard of care we're providing and improve where necessary. We can identify patients whose sugar control is poor, and redouble our efforts to help them. We can set alerts on our computer system to make sure checks and monitoring don't get overlooked and forgotten.

The register is also a bad thing. By coding Marta in this way, I was starting to push her down the route of having her metabolic problems medicalised. That need not be the case, of course. I am her doctor, after all, I can keep her situation under review. I can make judgements as to whether and when to offer medications, how long to give her to think about trying to tackle the problem in a different way. And were she to decide to give that approach a concerted go, I can monitor progress and see if we can achieve remission.

Well, that ought to be the case. And it would be were it just Marta and me alone in the consultation. But since 2004, there has been a third presence in the room. In 2004, the time-honoured two-way relationship between doctor and patient became, for the first time in medical history, a ménage à trois.

Like all such unconventional relationship set-ups, it started out seeming like a good idea. During the late 1990s, the government started to produce documents called National Service Frameworks (NSFs). Until that point, medical professionals had been responsible for ensuring their practice remained up-to-date. Most did this assiduously but some did not – remember the impressive but far from universal uptake of anti-clotting treatment for heart attacks that followed publication of the ISIS-2 trial. The seductive certainties growing out of the evidence-based medicine (EBM) movement proved irresistible to government, concerned by what were undoubtedly variations in standards of care. NSFs were its first response.

NSFs were based on the latest evidence and set out gold standards for care in conditions such as diabetes or heart disease. In effect, they built on the initiative of the Cochrane Collaboration, which we met in the last chapter. But while the Cochrane Reviews were put out there to be found by interested clinicians, NSFs were sent to all general practices and relevant specialists, in effect saying: this is what you should be doing. They were the first iterations of what would evolve into today's guideline culture.

Crucially, though, NSFs were what one would ideally aim for, but doctors were free to adapt them in light of each patient's situation. In 2004, however, as part of a major new contract for general practice, NSFs morphed into the Quality and Outcomes Framework (QOF). Instead of NSFs being advisory tools to help practices monitor and raise standards of care, QOF set targets – the percentage of diabetics with HbA1c results below a certain level, what proportion of patients we'd managed to get on a statin, and so on – and rewarded practices that achieved them with handsome bonus payments. To begin with, GPs welcomed the new system. The vast majority were already providing standards of care above the government targets so QOF brought a welcome influx of money into their practices, boosting income substantially. We will not have been the first group of people in history to have been so seduced by the silver being pressed into our palms that we didn't appreciate the downsides. In the years since QOF was first established, it has lost ever more favour with the profession, and is now widely despised. Through the exercise of financial levers government is, for the first time in medical history, micromanaging what doctors do clinically day to day. And it's not just micro-management, it is micromanagement down very narrow, disease-model pathways.

In coding Marta as a type 2 diabetic, I was entering her in our QOF. At year-end, were her HbA1c to be above the stipulated target figure, she would count as a black mark against us. There was now a vested interest within the practice in getting her control swiftly established. Weight loss, exercise and dietary change all take time. Drugs work much faster. The pressure to prescribe is considerable.

Of course, one could always initiate drug treatment to bring down the HbA1c while simultaneously encouraging lifestyle change, but that is a real mix of messages. Subliminally, one is saying two contradictory things: you can sort this out yourself, reverse the situation, but at the same time you need the paraphernalia of modern medicine to do it for you. The latter undermines the former. When faced with day-to-day decisions to change the eating habits of a lifetime, the notion in the back of the mind that there are pills that can make it all OK inevitably weakens resolve.

I closed down Marta's record and turned to the notes for my next patient. It would be another three months before I saw her again. We would pick up the threads then.

—

The first hurdle David Unwin encountered in trying to do something different about type 2 diabetes was his own colleagues, the partners in his practice. When he went to them and outlined his plan to offer type 2 diabetic patients the chance to try to reverse their condition through a low-carb diet, he met with flat refusal. 'We weren't paid [by QOF] to do that kind of work in 2012,' he explained. It would take up consultation time that would otherwise be used for activity that generated income for the surgery. And if his patients failed to demonstrate improvement or took too long to achieve it (and remember, none of his colleagues back then would have believed type 2 diabetes could be reversed) then the practice would suffer financial penalties.

Unwin was not put off. He started to work with type 2 diabetic patients in his own time, meeting groups of them on Monday evenings. He was joined by one of his practice nurses who, inspired by his enthusiasm and vision, offered to help unpaid. Unwin's wife, a practising psychologist, also volunteered for the project, bringing her expertise to bear in how best to motivate and maintain behavioural change.

It wasn't long before their first successes. Unwin collected data on every patient, charting their weight loss, the reductions they were achieving in HbA1c, and simultaneously finding he was tracking improvements in high blood pressure and blood cholesterol profiles to boot. He showed me a number of before-and-after photos, the smiles of visibly trimmer patients conveying the human face of the metabolic improvements their bodies were undergoing. Not every patient managed meaningful change, but there were enough dramatic outcomes – patients who had been type 2 diabetic for years coming off all treatment and maintaining normal HbA1cs – to convince his previously sceptical partners. Before long, the whole practice was adopting a low-carb approach.

Unwin started to write up his findings, publishing papers detailing the remarkable results he was achieving. In 2016 he joined forces with a number of other like-minded physicians to found the Public Health Collaboration, a charity dedicated to improving public health and simultaneously saving the NHS money through the provision of better lifestyle information. Unwin began working with diabetes.co.uk to formalise a low-carb diet plan, creating graphics to inform about the sugar content of various foodstuffs (150g of basmati rice, for example, contains the equivalent of ten teaspoonsful).

To him, what he was doing made perfect sense. Type 2 diabetes reflected slow poisoning by excessive sugar, so logically the thing to do was to scale the intake right back – exactly the approach one would take with a patient with coeliac disease whose body was being damaged by exposure to gluten, or a heavy drinker whose liver was showing signs of strain. The disease model we had all been trained to follow in type 2 diabetes was merely mitigating the harms, not getting to the cause. And in fact, many of the drugs we use, including insulin, compound the situation. Buried in the fine detail of the UK Prospective Diabetes Study was the awkward truth that, in lowering blood sugar levels, several of our pharmaceutical agents promote additional fat formation, further choking the liver and pancreas. Doctors were unwittingly enrolling type 2 diabetic patients in a downward spiral.

If Unwin expected plaudits for his work, he was soon disabused. New thinking is often intensely threatening to those whose long-held beliefs it undermines. For a number of years, the British Diabetic Association fought against the whole notion that the condition could be reversed (they eventually changed their position). Just as unexpectedly, Unwin's low-carb approach met fierce resistance from professional dieticians – to the extent that Unwin would receive what he describes as 'hate mail' from certain professionals. It wasn't just that they were sceptical about his claims; they thought his low-carb diet to be intrinsically dangerous. Think back to that exhibition room at my medical school library, the coronary artery becoming blocked by cholesterol-laden plaque. Since the early 1980s, the thrust of dietary advice has been to reduce the amount of saturated fat and cholesterol we eat, on the simplistic assumption that what goes in our mouths gets deposited in arterial walls. But eating less fat (together with the protein that is so frequently bound up alongside it) creates a calorie gap. Carbohydrates were seen as a harmless, even healthy way of replacing this missing energy. Unwin's low-carb approach tilts the balance back the other way. The dietician community feared high-protein intake would damage kidneys (Unwin has shown that it doesn't), and that a move away from 'low fat' products (which incidentally are frequently high in carbohydrate) would cause more heart disease. The evidence for that is surprisingly mixed and probably says more about the limitations of research methodology than anything else. What we do know is that type 2 diabetes greatly increases the risk of heart disease, and it is carbohydrate, not fat, that is the dietary driver for developing the condition.

Unwin was undeterred by the flak. He was sure he was onto something important. The calories contained in protein and fat don't provoke significant insulin secretion, hence are much less likely to stimulate the deposition of fat in the liver and pancreas that causes most type 2 diabetes. And calorie-for-calorie, protein and fat promote early satiety, reducing overall food intake by swiftly making people feel full. Carbohydrate on the other hand triggers insulin release – and rapid surges of sugar create hunger pangs as they are cleared from the bloodstream, encouraging further appetite. There are several factors behind the epidemic of type 2 diabetes that has swamped our society, including our increasingly sedentary lifestyles. But the anti-fat, pro-carbohydrate diet that has dominated health advice for the past forty years is arguably one of the most important.

—

No one is ever in any doubt, if they see Matilde and Marta together, that they are mother and daughter. They have the same thick black hair with a hint of a wave. Their heart-shaped faces and olive complexions are identical. And they regard the world through equally striking dark brown eyes. Matilde's, like her daughter's, are slightly magnified behind large-framed glasses. They remind me of a couple of those nested matryoshka dolls, carbon copies of one another except for being slightly different sizes (Marta is the taller).

I looked at the pair of them, sitting side by side in my consulting room just a couple of weeks after I gave Marta her diagnosis. 'How can I help?'

The appointment had been made for Matilde; Marta was here in her usual support role. Matilde reached into her handbag and extracted a bit of paper, which I instantly recognised as my rough guide to diabetes.

'I do not like these injections. I hate them,' Matilde said. The word hate was issued with suitable venom. 'Marta says perhaps I will not need them.'

She closed the clasp on the top of her handbag and held the diagram out to me, giving it a flourish. I wasn't entirely sure I needed it back, but I took it just the same. I was surprised by the turn of events. At the time, Marta hadn't looked like she'd given my talk much credence, but it seemed she'd gone straight home and discussed it with her mum. I glanced at her. Her expression was unreadable.

'OK, yes. Well, shall I talk you through it as well?'

I went through the basics just as I had done with Marta, this time trying to add a simplified explanation of the vicious circle Matilde was trapped in. How the more tablets and injections we had to use to reduce her sugar levels, the more that prompted her body to turn the excess sugar into fat. And how that fat then further blunted the insulin from working properly. So the more her sugar levels tended to rise.

I paused periodically, trying to gauge her understanding. Marta herself evidently thought Matilde couldn't be following me, she turned to her mum at one point and started talking rapidly in Portuguese. I didn't understand the words but the tone was unmistakable; there was exasperation there.

I was conscious of a vague bubbling of panic. Since becoming aware of David Unwin's work, I'd explained the low-carb approach to a couple of newly diagnosed type 2 diabetics, and a handful of others whose blood tests suggested they were heading that way. I'd had two definite successes. But I had only ever introduced it to people in the very earliest stages of the condition, patients either not on any medication or at most taking nothing but metformin, the oldest and least problematic of our diabetes drugs. I had nothing like Unwin's level of expertise. The prospect of trying to support a patient like Matilde, so many years down the line, whose pancreas was so exhausted that she needed her insulin topped up by injection, felt daunting. I wasn't at all sure her condition would even be reversible. There is thought to be a point of no return, a stage when the pancreas is so depleted that patients will depend on insulin therapy for the rest of their lives.

Even were Matilde not to have reached that Rubicon, my mind was buzzing with anticipatory problems. Were she to dramatically cut back on the hidden sugars in her diet, her current treatment would need to be reduced in advance, otherwise I would create a different sort of problem, dropping her blood sugars too low: hypoglycaemia. I felt distinctly out of my depth. It was not something I'd handled before. And I was acutely aware that my dietary advice was very broad brushstroke, that I lacked detailed knowledge. While in some parts of the country local NHS commissioners are funding patients to enrol on diabetes.co.uk's Low Carb Program (the fruits of David Unwin's collaboration with the charity), the funding is not available in my area. The NHS has in recent years woken up to the importance of weight loss – indeed, QOF now incentivises me to send newly diagnosed patients like Marta to an education programme supposed to encourage lifestyle change – but it remains stuck in the past. Were I to refer Matilde to a dietician, she would be coached in a calorie-restricted diet, but it would still be one that encouraged starchy carbohydrates as the principal source of energy. Contradictory messages from two different professionals.

Matilde listened to her daughter's translation, her gaze fixed somewhere across the room, her head occasionally nodding. At the end of Marta's spiel, Matilde gave a single, emphatic nod and looked directly at me. 'This is something I would very much like.'

I had clearly set wheels in motion that I hadn't intended, and it was time to come clean. I explained my limited experience with this new approach, the potential pitfalls along the way and apologised if I had inadvertently raised expectations.

But Matilde was evidently resolved and brushed aside my hesitations. I got a sudden appreciation of the grit that had seen her up sticks and move to a completely different country when her daughter's life had fallen apart.

Fortunately, being on insulin treatment, she was already well-versed in home-testing her blood sugars so would be able to monitor for low levels. And although I wasn't going to be able to get direct support from a dietician locally, Unwin's Public Health Collaboration has made a wealth of information about a low-carb diet available free of charge online. I also pointed her in the direction of diabetes.co.uk, where there are plentiful resources, including paid access to the Low Carb Program. We agreed that she would go home and, with Marta's support, do more reading and preparation. If she remained determined to embark on this course, she would come back and we would plan an initial reduction in her insulin treatment to give her suitable headroom.

She left looking satisfied, pausing only to retrieve the diagram I now somewhat regretted ever having drawn. She folded it crisply and stowed it back in her handbag. Marta got up to follow her. She gave me a smile that got nowhere near her eyes.

—

David Unwin's pioneering work has transformed his life. He still looks disbelieving as he recaps his achievements: from being a burned-out, fifty-five-year-old 'completely ordinary GP', he is, at the age of sixty-three, 'the happiest doctor I know'. He has published seventeen academic papers demonstrating the success of his low-carb approach and is in high demand as a speaker and educator. He holds a clutch of national appointments advising and influencing professional policy. The Low Carb Program he devised jointly with diabetes.co.uk has been used by nearly half a million people worldwide to date. Closer to home, his Southport practice has reversed the diabetes of nearly a quarter of their total type 2 diabetic population – 114 patients and counting. They calculate they're saving the NHS £68,000 annually on diabetic drugs alone – to say nothing of the costs of avoided complications, medical investigations and clinician time.

Aside from all that, Unwin has rediscovered the joy of medicine. 'For me, being a doctor is about using my skills and experience to make a difference.' He is keen to emphasise that he is far from starry-eyed; not everyone achieves remission through the low-carb approach and he still employs drugs where required. And every patient who reverses their condition still needs an annual HbA1c to ensure they remain controlled. Inevitably, maintenance is sometimes a problem. Unwin showed me a graph of one of his male patients, the HbA1c gradually creeping back up into the diabetic range a few years following reversal. But even this apparent relapse provoked a positive response: 'Most clinicians seeing that would say, right, it's time to add a drug back in.' Unwin instead reflected back to the relapsed patient that their blood results indicated that their carbohydrate load had increased. It proved to be enough. The graph for the same patient showed his sugar control coming back to normal following a restoration of his previous dietary habits. Unwin has given, and continues to give, so many patients hope.

Unwin is not the only person to be changing our understanding of type 2 diabetes, and the low-carb approach is not the only game in town. Weight loss achieved by any means can bring the condition into remission. And since 2014, evidence has been emerging of the disturbing effects of the chemically manipulated compounds introduced into ultra-processed foods (UPFs) to render them palatable and 'moreish'. UPFs now constitute the largest part of the typical British (and American) diet, and they appear to drive excess calorie consumption through the same brain pathways that underlie addiction. The role of the food industry in driving the obesity epidemic is becoming ever more plain.

But Unwin's story casts a light on much that ails medicine, too. Pioneering as he undoubtedly is, Unwin has merely rediscovered something that was once taken as read. Although therapeutic insulin – essential to the treatment of type 1 diabetes – began to be used in the 1920s, it wasn't until the late 1950s that the first tablet treatments were developed for type 2 diabetes. Their use didn't become widespread in the UK until the 1970s. Prior to that, doctors routinely prescribed low-carbohydrate diets to their diabetic patients, that being the only thing they could do to help keep them well – something that became lost with the passing of a generation.

How have we turned what is a social, environmental, commercial and cultural issue into a purely medical one? First drugs were developed to improve the lot of type 2 diabetic patients, which can only have seemed a good thing at the time. But gradually, the availability of pharmaceutical interventions allowed a disease model to take hold, doctors assumed control of the condition, and the crucial importance of dietary factors began to fade. The advent of EBM accelerated this process. Since the pharmaceutical industry funds the vast majority of clinical trials, the evidence on which we base our practice is unremittingly drug-focused. And the lure of new profits drives further research and development. The past twenty years have seen a slew of new classes of pharmaceuticals all capable of lowering HbA1c. Patients are prescribed more and more agents to hold their sugar levels down. It will surprise you to learn that few have actually been shown to improve clinical outcomes. If a drug can be demonstrated to lower HbA1c it has to be good, that is the assumption. We have touched on the role some drugs play in accelerating weight gain; others have been withdrawn because of causing unacceptable harm. In trials that have been quietly sidelined, too aggressive an approach to pharmaceutical lowering of HbA1c was found to increase mortality. Drugs are never an unalloyed good. Using them complacently, cavalierly, has distracted doctors from providing a holistic approach that would serve their patients so much better.

The medical profession bears significant responsibility for this state of affairs, but government has played a substantial role. The concept of type 2 diabetes as a disease has been rendered concrete by the ménage à trois of patient, doctor and QOF – we are paid to treat it this way and penalised if we do not. With millions nationwide now suffering the effects of sugar poisoning, it is estimated by Diabetes UK that as much as 10% of the entire NHS budget is spent in managing the condition. The sheer scale of the effort – identifying cases, prescribing drugs, monitoring control, screening for complications, treating them when they occur – is gargantuan. Even though the NHS is gradually waking up to the potential to prevent and reverse the condition, this represents still more demand on our overloaded health service.

The explosion in type 2 diabetes over the past few decades has its genesis in population factors – the kinds of food available to us, the kinds of foods we think we should eat, our sedentary lifestyles, together with socioeconomic adversity and poverty which have been shown time and again to be a barrier to healthy lifestyle choices. These kinds of factors are amenable to policy action, yet public health has been progressively eroded as a force in the UK over the past twenty years. It runs counter to the currently prevailing culture of our politics, where levers such as an effective sugar tax and advertising prohibitions are deemed 'nannying', and policies to seriously address the deprivation that helps drive unhealthy nutrition and lifestyles are the stuff of never-never land. Beneath these factors lurks the baleful influence of corporate lobbying, both from a food industry wanting to avoid scrutiny and additional regulation, and from a pharmaceutical industry profiting handsomely from the medicalisation of lifestyle 'disease'.

It is far more convenient to all these interests if type 2 diabetes is a disease, and if responsibility for it is located with the individual. It is then up to the health service to pick up the pieces. We need instead to face up to the fact that the epidemic of type 2 diabetes is telling us we have a huge public health problem, something that government, through revitalised public health policies, has a critical role in helping to solve.

We've done this before. In the 1960s around two-thirds of adults smoked, an activity that was widely considered normal. Today, smoking prevalence is around 15%. The NHS has played a part in this. Brief advice to quit from a trusted GP has been shown to be one of the most potent interventions for catalysing change, and the provision of smoking cessation services has been one of the NHS's most cost-effective activities, helping to prevent countless cases of cancer, respiratory and heart disease. But the health service's efforts have been embedded within a far wider public health approach, including taxation policy, restriction on advertising and packaging, public information campaigns and legislative manoeuvres to progressively banish smoking from public and indoor spaces, all of which have turned what was once considered normal into something borderline socially unacceptable. Another key lesson from tackling tobacco is that industry will only make meaningful changes when forced to do so by policy and legislation.

—

Marta is, in many ways, fortunate. Matilde collects the boys at the end of the school day and looks after them in holidays, so Marta can work without having to constantly juggle childcare considerations. When she returns home at the end of the day, her mum has already attended to any number of household tasks that would otherwise sap her remaining time and energy. Were she motivated to try to reverse her type 2 diabetes she would be a great deal better placed than many, for whom convenience foods and snacks are a lifeline amid the unrelenting pressures of 'just about managing' life. But not for nothing do we have the phrase 'comfort food'.

Marta has wrestled with low mood since her marriage broke down. She came to the UK chasing a joint dream with her ex-husband, Salvador, and that has disintegrated. Faced with the choice between uprooting her children and returning home, or sticking it out in her adopted country, she elected to stay, only to run slap-bang into the poisonous impacts of Brexit and the waves of anti-immigrant sentiment that have swirled in its wake. I don't know if she wishes she could find a new partner or not, but in any event nothing has materialised to date. Matilde is, in all sorts of ways, her saving grace. I also wonder about the relationship between them. They generally come across congenially but there can be undercurrents. I imagine the role of the extended family remains stronger in Portuguese culture than in our own. Even so, I sometimes sense that Marta is frustrated by her enforced dependence on her mum, although she has never expressed that out loud to me.

Matilde concerns me far less. I have never been privy to the circumstances she left behind in Portugal, other than that she was widowed at a relatively young age, but she always strikes me as relishing the role of grandmother-in-residence and chief supporter of her divorced daughter. She possesses indefatigable energy and seems to thrive on keeping the family's domestic life shipshape.

One of her many roles is in sorting out the food shopping and preparing most of the meals. I know this because of the impact on her diabetes. Over the course of ten months or so, she managed to lose a stone and a half. It was my practice nurse who gave her the good news: her HbA1c remained well-controlled even without the quarter dose we'd finally brought her insulin down to. I saw her shortly afterwards about a mole on her cheek. It was obviously benign so after reassuring her I asked how she'd found adapting to a low-carb diet. She held a hand out and rocked it side to side in the time-honoured 'so-so' gesture. It was evidently taxing to think of the English to explain further, so she rapped out several sentences in her mother tongue.

'She says it got her back in touch with our traditional cooking, though she bakes and grills and doesn't do too much of the frying,' Marta translated. Then she added a sotto voce comment of her own. 'I can't tell you how much fish we're eating.'

Matilde laughed and put a hand on her daughter's hand. 'I am very happy I do not need injections any more.'

I don't know what the future will hold, whether she will continue to lose weight and see if she can do without her tablet treatments, too, or whether her personal goal was to get rid of insulin and she will be content now she's achieved that.

Marta got up from her chair, ready to go. 'You've done amazingly, as well,' I said to her. I'd checked up on her latest HbA1c before calling them through. Though still just in the 'borderline' category, she'd dropped right out of the diabetic range and had done so without ever requiring any drugs.

She rolled her eyes. 'Like I say, I can't tell you about all the fish.'

Matilde, too, had got to her feet. The skin round her eyes was still crinkled with amusement. As she followed her daughter out of the room she extended a hand towards me.

I think she was intending to clasp mine, or rest hers briefly on my arm, but if so she hesitated, perhaps wary that Marta might see. Instead she made a fist, which she used to give a triumphant little shake. It was exceptionally brief but when I met her gaze, I could have sworn she winked, too.

4

THE NATIONAL RISK SERVICE

Michael had come following an NHS health check. 'They said it was my cholesterol,' he told me as I showed him into my room. 'Is it very high?'

This is a widely held concern and almost entirely a myth. There are uncommon genetic disorders that lead to markedly raised cholesterol levels, which are in turn associated with early onset heart disease – the family history usually features several relatives who have suffered heart attacks in their forties or even younger. But for the vast majority of us, our cholesterol level viewed in isolation is essentially meaningless.

I sat myself down and called Michael's results up on the computer. 'Nothing dramatic,' I said. 'But it's not the absolute figure that matters, it's who's got it. Let me show you.'

With a couple more clicks, I pulled up something called a Qrisk calculator. I turned my screen slightly so Michael could see. 'This crunches all sorts of things about you – your age, sex, blood pressure, whether you smoke or have diabetes, that kind of thing. Then it interprets your cholesterol in light of all that.'

Michael shifted his chair and leaned in. I ran the programme. His risk estimate popped up in the middle of the screen: 12.14%. The figure was rendered in stark red, one of nature's clearest warning signals. It drew the eye compellingly.

'So that's saying: if you have a hundred identical Michaels with just that level of cholesterol, over the next decade twelve of you are likely to develop heart disease or have a stroke.' We sat in silence for a couple of seconds. 'Mind you, eighty-eight of you won't.' I could hear how limp my addendum sounded. Already Qrisk with its alarming colour scheme was emphasising the negative, the danger.

I know Michael through his family. His wife, Caroline, has had problems with depression stemming from experiences in foster care as a child. Their younger daughter, Olivia, has suffered a lot with abdominal problems. Michael, head of year at a nearby secondary school, has proved sensible and pragmatic as we've steered a delicate course, trying to ensure we're not missing something significant behind Olivia's symptoms while not losing sight of the likely causes: family dynamics and, in Olivia, an anxious predisposition.

Michael hardly ever consults about himself, though – vaccinations aside, the last time we'd seen him had been years before, when we'd arranged a vasectomy. In his early fifties, he's enjoyed robust good health throughout his adult life. Then he'd attended a health check at the invitation of the NHS, and now that Qrisk score had cast a shadow. Those stark red figures. One day, they seemed to be telling him, one day your sustained run of good luck is going to come to an end.

'So what do I do about that?' he said.

These kinds of discussions are complicated, becoming ever more so the deeper one delves. And because we're all human, one can never be sure exactly how they're going to turn out.

'Well, a lot of doctors would say you should take a statin,' I told him. 'You know what they are?'

'Drugs that lower cholesterol.'

I nodded. 'Drugs that lower cholesterol – and they'll definitely do that for you if you take them. They're also drugs that reduce the risk of heart disease. The two aren't necessarily as connected as you might think.' I clicked on a button on the Qrisk tool. 'Let's see what they might do for you.'

A new dialogue box opened up, filled with 100 hearts arranged in neat 10 x 10 rows. Almost all of them were pink. On the very bottom row, though, nine of the ten were shown in pillar box red, each sundered by a zigzag line down the middle.

'So, that's your one hundred Michaels,' I started to explain. 'Imagine I give you all a statin to take every day for the next ten years. After that, I invite you back for a reunion. There's going to be one or two who don't make it—' I pointed to the broken red hearts at the bottom of the chart '—and another seven or so who come back with stories about how they've developed angina or survived a heart attack. But ninety-one Michaels – almost all of you – are going to be there entirely unscathed.'

I let him digest the graphic for a moment or two. 'Remember, every one of these Michaels has been taking a statin every day for a decade. The only ones that got any benefit from it are these three.' There was a small white pill next to the final three of the ninety-one pink hearts, to indicate that the statin tablets had prevented them from turning red and breaking. 'Eighty-eight of you weren't going to get heart disease anyway. Nine of you developed it in spite of taking the statins. Only these three gained anything.'

I smiled wryly. 'If we knew which Michaels they were going to be, it would be easy. But we don't. So we end up having to treat all one hundred of you, and some of you will develop side effects along the way.'

I paused again; there was a lot to take in. I try to have these conversations with anyone eligible for primary prevention – people who are perfectly healthy but who are deemed at risk – but it can be quite a culture shock. Michael asked a couple of questions. He was struck by the legions of pink-hearted people who would remain well irrespective of whether they took statins. But he seemed positively disturbed by the fact that, of the dozen individuals fated to develop heart disease, the majority would still do so despite religiously taking preventative pills.

'I had absolutely no idea,' he said.

'You're in good company.'

Most people get their information about statins from the media, certain sections of which extol them in such glowing terms that they have achieved near elixir-of-life status. Equally, other sectors of the press present them entirely negatively, overemphasising their side effects and underplaying their role. Neither is right. They're modestly useful drugs for people like my guitar-playing patient Simon. Having survived a heart attack, he has revealed himself to be one of the unlucky broken-red-hearted ones, so would probably want to take a medication that might shave off some of the risk of a further episode, assuming he tolerated it OK. That's called secondary prevention – risk reduction in someone who's got established disease. I'd also be inclined to take one for primary prevention if I had the genes for pathologically raised cholesterol. That's the scenario where statins demonstrate the greatest impact. But for someone like Michael – fit and well and with a modest Qrisk: well, that's far more finely balanced.

'Not wanting to overcomplicate things,' I said, 'although statins make a difference to perhaps three of these hundred Michaels, there's huge debate over whether that actually results in any saved lives.'

This concept can be additionally confusing but it's important, so I tried my best to explain. Looked at narrowly in terms of cardiovascular disease, which is all that the pink heart/red heart graphic shows, statins appear to do a little bit of good. But many other things go wrong with us. Over the ten years of daily statin therapy illustrated, some of those 100 Michaels will develop cancer, others might meet with a fatal accident or overwhelming sepsis or die from cirrhosis, severe depression could lead another to suicide. The idea that all ninety-one pink-hearted Michaels would return for the reunion is false – some others wouldn't make it for unrelated reasons. If you consider all-cause mortality – deaths from any disease – the total numbers come out roughly the same. Put simply, perhaps one person in the hundred taking statins would avoid a fatal heart attack, but that might only allow them to die from something else. Statins for primary prevention may occasionally change the cause of death but they don't much alter the fact of it.

'Last thing, I promise.' I checked to see if Michael was still with me. He gave me a nod to go on. 'This chart is just about what happens with a statin. We don't have similar ones for alternatives. Exercise also reduces the chances of heart disease – more so, probably, than statins. And it benefits a whole load of other health problems, things like cancer risk, so it does reduce all-cause mortality.'

Michael nodded again. 'OK.'

There was an upward inflection on the 'K' – he wanted to hear more. I gave him details of a YouTube video called 'Twenty-three and a half hours' in which American physician Mike Evans rounds up the considerable but largely unappreciated evidence base for the beneficial health impact of even very modest amounts of non-Lycra exercise (brisk walking).

'It's not either/or,' I said. 'But the problem with stuff like this—' I waved a hand towards the computer screen '—is it makes us focus on drugs, and we might miss out on things that are a whole lot better for you. And in any case, Qrisk doesn't take any account of how much exercise you do, nor what kind of diet you eat.' I glanced back at the screen with its stark red 12.14%. 'It looks very precise, doesn't it, with those two decimal points? But it's only a rough guide. A very rough guide.'

Michael slapped both palms against his belly. 'I had been thinking about getting a bit more into shape.' He's not actually overweight but he'd evidently become aware of middle-aged spread. 'This might be the warning shot I needed. As for that, though,' he nodded towards the computer screen with its hundred-heart graphic about statins, 'thanks for talking me through it. But it doesn't look worth it to me.'

—

Doctors have always taken account of risk factors. Take a presenting symptom like chest pain. If the patient is a sixty-nine-year-old male smoker, with a history of diabetes and high blood pressure and a family history of heart disease, then the chance of his pain being cardiac in origin is pretty high. The same symptom in a thirty-four-year-old female account director, using the pill for contraception and just back from America where she was visiting her mother who was recovering from a deep vein thrombosis, is much more likely to represent a blood clot on the lungs. Coupled with features like the characteristics of the pain, risk factors help to narrow down the cause and guide investigation and treatment. For almost the entirety of medical history, the notion of risk has helped doctors in diagnosis – the process of working out what is actually wrong.

Prognosis – predicting the future – has also long been central to medicine. Having arrived at a diagnosis, what does the physician's knowledge and experience suggest is going to happen? Is this the sort of condition that should get better in time? Are there treatments that might help? If it can't be cured, what can the patient and their family expect? And in the toughest of scenarios: how long is there left to live?

These twin capabilities – diagnosis and prognosis – have been core to the art of medicine for centuries, not least in the era before doctors had effective treatments. Kenneth Lane, a GP who practised in the same town as me in the 1930s, well before the advent of antibiotics, described in his memoirs his intimate familiarity with the usual course of common, serious infectious diseases. In bacterial pneumonia, for example, there was a constellation of telltale signs around the eleventh day that allowed Lane to predict whether the patient was ultimately going to survive or die. Such soothsaying abilities have traditionally contributed substantially to the power and mystique of the doctor.

During the course of my career, medicine has been attempting to occupy a whole new territory, that of risk. The theory is seductive: if we can identify who is at high risk of developing a certain condition then it might be possible to prevent it happening. Superficially, it has much in common with those traditional arts, diagnosis and prognosis. But instead of diagnosing a disease, we are attempting to 'diagnose' someone's risk. And the physician's reputation for prowess in prognosis endows such risk assessments with a quality of near inevitability. If a doctor tells you you are at risk of developing a certain condition, it can feel like they are foretelling your future.

We are actually very poor at it. Those same risk factors that prove so useful when arriving at a diagnosis – demographics like age and sex, lifestyle factors like smoking and exercise, biological markers such as blood pressure, weight, glucose and cholesterol – provide very poor predictive power. We dress them up pseudoscientifically – expressing them to two decimal places, colour-coding them to lend them a weight they don't deserve. But neither our 'risk diagnoses' nor our recommendations for 'treatment' have any real application to the individual in front of us.

Few people appreciate how different the NRS – the National Risk Service – is from the NHS. Most patients' ideas about doctors still reflect a world that medicine left behind a long time ago: an era when you went to the GP when you felt unwell, and when you fondly imagined that any treatment recommended would be highly likely to do you some good. 'You are at risk of heart disease' sounds like one day you are definitely going to come a cropper. And the prescription of a 'treatment' – take these statin tablets – feels like a continuation of what doctors have always done. Little wonder that, when asked in surveys, uninformed patients wildly overestimate their potential for benefit from a statin. When, like Michael, they learn that their chances of getting anything from taking it are marginal at best – 3% in his case – it can come as a significant shock.

Just as most patients have little understanding of the realities of the world of medical risk management, neither do many doctors. Like frogs in steadily heating water, as a profession we have no real appreciation of how far we have gone in conflating risk with disease. Our guidelines tell us to prescribe treatment X in the face of risk level Y, and QOF further incentivises this behaviour. As a consequence, we have around 8 million people taking statins in the UK, the majority for primary prevention. Most will have been simply handed a prescription and advised to take them, and will have no idea how marginal the benefits are. Only a small minority – studies suggest as few as 20% – will have encountered doctors with the information, training, time and confidence to have even attempted to have had an informed consent discussion.

How did we get here? At its heart lies the difference between the population and the personal. Imagine, for a moment, you're looking down on the UK from a very great height – from a satellite, say. You can't see individual people, all you have is an impression of millions of humans making up an entire population. Suppose you're aware that heart disease is a common problem, and that by getting everyone to take a daily pill you should be able to 'save' thousands of lives (leave aside for a moment the controversy about that claim). Then it becomes a question of how to get the statins into people. You could, perhaps, put them in the water, like fluoride, but that would court controversy. Or you could get your health service to try to pick out the people at highest risk and prescribe statins to them. No matter that our ability to diagnose risk is so poor. No matter that the vast majority will be taking drugs that won't benefit them. That feels like it must be a price worth paying for the lives 'saved'.

Now zoom right into the level of the individual, someone like Michael. If, in blissful ignorance, he believes there's a high chance the tablets he's being advised to take will help him, he's reasonably likely to go along with it (even then, though, if Michael is among the solid majority of people who are chary of the use of drugs, he may decide to pass). But if he gets given realistic information – which he needs in order to give informed consent to the 'treatment' – he may very well reject the idea of taking a pharmaceutical preparation every day for decades on the minute chance it might do him some good. Now multiply that by millions of Michaels across the country. Suddenly that vision – that by mass medicating a substantial proportion of the population you will reduce the burden of heart disease – begins to unravel.

Not that every individual will come to the same conclusion as Michael. I have had the exact same discussion with similar patients who do decide to embark on long-term statin treatment. Perception of risk varies enormously from person to person, and will be affected by all manner of factors. Someone who lost a close friend to heart disease might be more inclined to do anything they can to lower their own chances of suffering a similar fate. And locus of control is also important. People with a strong internal locus of control believe they can take charge and change their own future, others with a strong external locus believe they are essentially at the mercy of events and will be more inclined to accept outside help. These kinds of factors combine to form an individual's 'health beliefs', which are a powerful determinant when making decisions about medical matters. But my personal experience of having conducted numerous informed consent discussions about primary prevention suggest to me that the large majority of people will decline long-term drugs that have a very low prospect of doing them good.

—

Caroline had to help Michael on the walk from the waiting room.

'Take your time,' I said, trying to counter any sense that they had to hurry. Even though his wife was supporting much of his weight, Michael winced every time his right leg was in contact with the ground.

'What happened?' I asked, once we'd made it inside my consulting room and Michael had been safely installed on a chair.

He gave a rueful smile. 'As soon as I got back from seeing you, I went and dug out my old trainers and running gear. Strike while the iron's hot!' His chuckle was suffused with irony. 'I'd got halfway round the field behind the house when I landed my foot in a hole.'

His ankle was less swollen than I'd have expected. As I

examined it, something very odd came to light. The long tendon that normally wraps behind the bony prominence on the outside of the ankle was displaced forwards, essentially flapping free from its moorings.

'I think we'd better get you seen at fracture clinic,' I said. 'Not that you've broken anything. But you've completely torn the ligament at the side here, look.'

Most ankle sprains heal up without the need for intervention, but Michael's was of a different order. He had six weeks in a cast and on crutches but even that failed to restore the strength and stability. Ultimately he had to have surgery to repair the fibrous tissue that holds the tendon in place. It was many months before he could think of exercising again, and running remains firmly off the agenda.

One-off cases shouldn't sway practice, but Michael's almost farcical return to athletic endeavour was an impressive example of the law of unintended consequences. Reflecting on it, I kept coming back to those stark red figures: 12.14%. One day, they seemed to say, one day your sustained run of good luck is going to come to an end. And of course that is true for all of us. But Qrisk's colour-coded warning was far from as straightforward as it appeared. Had Michael and I had the same conversation, using the exact same tool prior to 2015, that 12.14% would have been presented in plain black. Nothing to see here. Nothing to worry about. Until that point, Qrisk would turn its risk prediction figure red only once a 20% threshold had been reached. What had changed in 2015 to turn someone like Michael from a carefree individual into someone deemed 'at risk' of heart disease?

The simple answer is the cost of statins. When a drug comes off patent – which in practical terms is usually around ten years after coming on the market – the company that developed it loses its exclusive rights. Competitor companies launch rival products, called generics, and purchasing costs to the NHS typically tumble. When developing its guidelines, NICE takes a narrowly economic view: if a patented drug could be used for primary prevention, the costs generally constrain its use to the highest-risk patients – those who, statistically speaking, stand the most chance of gain. Once cheap generics become available, the economics change, and it becomes affordable to recommend the medication be used at ever lower levels of risk. This leads to ever greater numbers of people being scooped up into the medicalisation net. When NICE lowered its risk threshold from 20% to 10% in 2015, they rendered an additional 4.5 million adults in the UK eligible for primary prevention. Just like Michael's 12.14%, 4.5 million adults' Qrisk predictions turned from reassuring black to alarm-bell red overnight.

This mass medication strategy, that seems to make such sense from a population perspective, has a huge impact on the NHS, with vast numbers of people turned into patients, undergoing blood tests and consultations and consuming millions of tablets. And it will have knock-on effects for many. Yes there will be instances of heart disease and stroke avoided, but are we in large part altering cause, not fact, of death? Then there is the burden of side effects. That question is as hotly contested as the level of benefit. Muscle pain is the commonest reason for people to discontinue taking statins, and as a subjective symptom it can also reflect many other things. The more evangelical the proponent of the mass medication strategy, the more likely they are to discount patients' experiences of adverse drug effects – to the extent that we now have the unedifying spectacle of academic papers exhorting doctors to disbelieve what their patients are telling them. Then there is that subtle but highly important psychological effect from the notion that there is a pill taking care of us: how much does that diminish some people's motivation to take care of themselves? If we're taking something we believe to be effective at protecting us from harm, does the sense of invulnerability affect the lifestyle choices we might otherwise take more note of?

Michael's unfortunate ankle injury – as isolated an event as it was – serves as a useful metaphor for these conundrums. Primary prevention is often presented as an unequivocal good. But there is no such thing as a one-sided coin.

—

Trefor was worried about prostate cancer. It wasn't that he had any symptoms – he felt fine and had no problems with the way his bladder was working. Nor was it something running rife in his family history. It was all the stuff in the media.

'I keep reading things about it in the paper. Then the other day there was this chap on the radio saying men of my age should go and get a PSA test. I thought I'd better come down.'

Prostate cancer is common – around 1 in 8 men will develop it over the course of a lifetime. A chemical called PSA will often be raised in the bloodstream when someone has the disease. It therefore seems perfectly logical to measure PSA as a way of trying pick up an unsuspected tumour. And perfectly logical that, if there proves to be one, doctors should crack on and operate on it or do some form of treatment, because it seems a *sine qua non* to get rid of a cancer at the earliest opportunity in order to try to effect a cure.

That's certainly the story that gets promulgated by certain influential celebrities who have themselves been diagnosed with the disease. And it's also the tacit message in much of the information put out by the charity Prostate Cancer UK. To someone like Trefor, encountering this kind of publicity in the course of everyday life, it can feel like he must be missing out on something important. Prostate Cancer UK has emulated the highly successful campaign surrounding the issue of breast cancer, creating a specially designed lapel badge with which to declare affiliation with the cause, and posting pictures of cheerful fundraisers wearing branded T-shirts on a 'March for Men'. And everyone knows about breast cancer screening using mammograms, to which all eligible women are invited. How much simpler it ought to be to screen men for prostate cancer with a blood test.

Only there's currently no national screening programme. That's not because of some bias against or neglect of men's health problems. The issue has been looked at in multiple studies and scrutinised by the UK national screening committee. It's because prostate cancer screening with PSA doesn't work.

How to approach this paradox with Trefor? He was looking at me expectantly.

'We can certainly measure your PSA if you decide you want to.' I'd been about to use the word 'check' but instead chose the more neutral 'measure'. 'But it's not as straightforward as you might have been led to believe. Do you know anything about the ins and outs?'

'Not really, no.'

There was a note of perplexity in his voice – this evidently wasn't quite the response he'd expected. I sketched out the most important points. How PSA is a lousy test – PSA is often raised for innocent reasons, and sometimes normal when prostate cancer is there. How, in trying to sort out what a raised PSA actually means, we end up subjecting a lot of men to invasive and sometimes harmful tests like biopsies taken through the rectum. And if we measured PSA systematically as part of a formal screening programme, we would end up detecting around twenty extra cases of prostate cancer in every thousand men, but we wouldn't save a single life by doing so. That's the most counter-intuitive thing: the extra prostate cancers identified via PSA screening would all be indolent – they would never have progressed to cause clinical disease. PSA screening would actually lead to more harm through the side effects of treatment – including incontinence and impotence, to say nothing of the anxiety of becoming a cancer patient – given for tumours that were never going to cause problems.

'So why did they say all that stuff on the radio?' Trefor asked.

I was pretty sure I knew which celebrity he'd heard – someone who had been nudged by a friend to have a PSA test, which had ultimately led to a cancer being diagnosed and excised. 'I guess it depends which end of the telescope you're looking through,' I said. 'If you have a test and it finds a tumour and you then have an operation and someone tells you your cancer's all gone, you're going to feel extremely lucky and grateful. It won't matter what the statistics say. To you, you've had cancer and a blood test led to it being picked up and cured. Of course you're going to go around telling others to do the same thing.'

Trefor looked thoughtful, perhaps imagining himself in that person's shoes. 'But there's not much point?'

'That's what the data show. But it's completely up to you – we can if you want. I just need you to know the facts so you can make an informed choice.'

He left with a copy of a leaflet that summarised the issues and promised to get back in touch if he decided to go ahead – though he thought he was unlikely to.

As I wrote up the notes, I was aware of a faint disquiet. I often get it after these kinds of discussions. A juju feeling – as though, by deciding against investigation, Trefor had tempted fate. I know colleagues who wouldn't have even attempted to discuss it – who, faced with someone like Trefor, would uncritically go along with ordering the test. They would reckon they're on a hiding to nothing were they to do otherwise. If you do a PSA and it's normal, the patient will be happy and grateful. If it subsequently transpires to have been a false negative and they later present with prostate cancer, at least they will be able to say, albeit with puzzled disbelief: 'My doctor even tested for it and it came back clear.' And if you get a raised PSA that, after weeks of uncertainty and further evaluation, turns out to be a false positive, then there's celebration and relief. If a cancer is found, though, then the patient enters the same narrative as the celebrity Trefor had heard speaking on the radio, one in which their cancer has been serendipitously detected, apparently giving them the very best shot at a cure.

I understand colleagues who take this quick and easy path but to me if feels deceptive. In every one of those scenarios, the doctor comes out the good guy. Yet the anxiety and discomfort endured during evaluation of false positives, to say nothing of the 2% of men whom testing turns into cancer patients yet whose tumours would never have caused any problems – all these harms arise from clinicians not doing their job properly.

Sitting in the opposite chair, I would want someone to give me the information to make an informed choice. Then it would be down to me. If I went along a certain course of action and suffered foreseeable harm as a result, then that would have been my decision. And it might have been a risk I considered worth taking; that would depend on my health beliefs. But the key thing is: I would have been in charge.

Was that what I had done for Trefor, though? Had I presented things neutrally and allowed him to reach his own conclusion? Or had my own opinion – that PSA screening causes harm – coloured both the substance of what I'd said and the manner in which I'd said it? My view is derived from an objective look at population-level data and, certainly at the moment, I have no worries that I personally might be affected by the disease. But someone who is very anxious about the possibility might prefer to investigate, hoping for the reassurance a negative result would bring – even though it could be wrong – rather than living any longer with the apprehension and fear. Should I have spent a bit more time getting to the bottom of Trefor's concerns?

I gave myself a metaphorical shake to dispel the superstition. All I was doing was spooking myself. I couldn't imagine I had swayed Trefor in a way he might someday look back on and regret.

—

Screening is the other facet of the National Risk Service. There are a number of national programmes. The oldest is cervical screening, which, rather than detecting established cancer, seeks out cell changes that might, over a period of years, turn malignant. In this respect, the cervical smear test is a special case somewhat akin to Qrisk – it identifies women at high risk and provides treatment, albeit that the treatment for cervical changes is highly effective rather than marginal, destroying as it does the altered cells. Even allowing for the proportion of women who won't engage with what is, after all, a highly intimate investigation, the smear campaign is estimated to prevent around 70% of deaths from the disease.

There are some downsides – many more women are treated than would actually develop cancer, and occasionally, a treated cervix may not function properly in a subsequent pregnancy, for example – but taken as a whole, the programme is probably the best example of a successful screening initiative. (The advent of vaccination against the virus which causes virtually all cases of cervical cancer, HPV, looks like it will reduce the need for screening down to a single smear for most women, such is its efficacy in reducing the incidence of pre-cancerous change.)

The other national screening programmes are different, aiming to detect established cancer at an early, more readily curable stage. When the first of these – breast cancer screening – was instituted, it looked to be a similarly unalloyed good. Yes, the test – breast X-ray with mammography – was also intimate and uncomfortable, but the early trials suggested the programme was picking up many more cancers at an earlier stage and improving patients' chances of survival. As more data have emerged, however, the picture has become more complex. For every woman whose life is saved by undergoing screening, another three women will be diagnosed with cancer unnecessarily – a phenomenon called overdiagnosis. Until twenty years ago, our experience of the disease was based on cancers that present with clinical symptoms, and those malignancies very often behave aggressively and cause disability and death. What screening has revealed is that many other people develop tumours that will never progress to clinical disease. Bizarre as it may sound, cancer can sometimes be harmless.

Screening picks up both types of tumour: those that will progress to disease and those that won't. And the problem is, we don't yet know how to tell them apart. The only solution at present is to treat all cancers as potentially injurious – hence the significant numbers of screened women who will undergo surgery, radiotherapy, chemotherapy and hormone treatment unnecessarily.

It took considerable effort on the part of campaigners to have this information made available to women invited for mammography. It was feared that faced with such concrete downsides to screening, many women would opt out, reducing the effectiveness of the programme. Akin to the mass medication scenario with statins, 'population' thinking was felt to trump the 'personal'. But the concept of informed consent is fundamental to medical practice, and the argument to provide unbiased information about the pros and cons of mammographic screening eventually prevailed. And interestingly, the concerns about the programme becoming eroded have not materialised. Even once provided with information about overdiagnosis and overtreatment, most women still opt to proceed with screening. In each individual's calculus, there are many different factors that influence risk decisions. As a life-threatening disease, breast cancer has high visibility and feels to be a far more significant health problem for women than heart disease, even though more women die from heart attacks than breast cancer each year. And the prospect of having a cancer treated unnecessarily just in case it were ultimately to prove life-threatening probably feels very different to taking long-term medication to marginally reduce the risk of something that may very well never occur.

Trefor's situation was even more complex. Use of PSA as a screening test for prostate cancer saves no lives at all and carries the certain risk of overdiagnosis and overtreatment. There is accordingly no screening programme. But that is an example of population-level thinking. And that is far from the only lens through which the world can be viewed.

—

Something about the urologist's letter snagged my attention. It's never great to learn that a patient has been diagnosed with cancer. The biopsies from the prostate tumour suggested it would have a relatively good prognosis – not the absolute best, but only two notches above that, so the outlook after treatment was still positive. But it wasn't the details of the case that were nagging at me. It was the patient's first name: Trefor.

I read through the details of the radiotherapy that had been decided on, and the hormone-blocking injections to try to ensure the cancer stayed away, but my concentration was awry. Trefor is the Welsh equivalent of Trevor, and as far as I knew the only person I'd ever met who'd been christened with it was a patient at the practice. Yet while the name was familiar, I couldn't picture the man or the context.

I called up his notes on the computer and scanned the recent entries. It turned out he'd been dealt with by Hugh, another of the GPs at the surgery. Trefor had complained of needing to get up to the loo several times a night and some difficulty getting his stream flowing. The symptoms had been going on for three months. Hugh had done exactly what was necessary: a urine sample had come back clear, rectal examination had been unremarkable, but the PSA in his blood test had proved to be raised. Hugh had organised an urgent referral under the 'two week wait' pathway, biopsies had confirmed the suspected diagnosis, and what would hopefully prove to be curative treatment was about to get underway.

I hadn't been involved at all.

I was curious now. I must have encountered Trefor at some point, but as I scanned back through the notes the only entries were from colleagues. Then suddenly there it was: my name at the head of an entry from two and a half years previously. I was right. I did know him.

It was a strange sensation, reading the notes I'd made back then. Trefor had come to discuss screening for prostate cancer. He'd been 'hearing a lot about it in the press, on the radio' – there was a celebrity, diagnosed with the disease following a PSA test, who'd been in the media urging men to 'get checked'.

My notes showed that Trefor had no urinary symptoms at the time. They recorded the salient details of the discussion, and the written information I'd provided. I had left it with him to decide whether he wanted to proceed.

I was struck by a sense of foreboding. Most cancers are present, silently growing, for years before reaching the stage of causing symptoms. Trefor's tumour may well have been there, unsuspected, at the time he had come to see me. If I had measured his PSA then, would it have been raised? Quite possibly, although I would never now know. I tried to quash my disquiet. Would Trefor remember our discussion? What would his recollections be? Had he felt he'd been given a genuine choice, or had my tone and demeanour communicated dismissiveness? His cancer now was of an intermediate grade, still likely to be curable, but how much more treatable might it have been had it been diagnosed those thirty months earlier?

I knew all the rational arguments, that at a population level PSA screening causes only harm. But how would they wash with Trefor now that his personal situation had crystallised in the most threatening way imaginable? I wouldn't have to wait long to find out. His computer records showed he had an appointment scheduled already for his first hormone-blocking injection. And the doctor he was booked in with was me. This could have been down to chance, I might have been the only one with an available appointment at the time the injection was due. Or it might have been a deliberate choice on his part – an opportunity for him to vent anger towards the GP he blamed for the diagnostic delay that had put him in a less favourable prognostic group.

I try always to be relaxed and friendly calling patients through from the waiting room – it's easy to become complacent dealing with dozens of people every day, but to each individual their visit to the doctor can be everything from routine to terrifying. He's a tall man, Trefor; he stands at least half a foot above me. He's in his early sixties, with a lanky build and a neat brown moustache. He makes me think of an army captain or brigadier, though he's never been in the military. I smiled as he crossed the waiting room, trying to read his body language to assess how the consultation was likely to be.

'I'm really sorry to hear the news,' I said, once we'd taken our seats. 'How are you doing?'

'I'm OK, actually,' he said. 'It was a shock. But the consultant was pretty upbeat. He thinks he should be able to deal with it OK.' He paused for a moment. 'Would you share that view?'

I talked him through the various bits of information – biopsy findings, scan results, PSA levels – and what they implied for his outlook. I was disarmed by his seeking my opinion about his prognosis. He certainly didn't come across as hostile or blaming. Perhaps our conversation those years before had even become lost to memory. I'd prepared the injection prior to calling him through so I proceeded to administer it, having run through the potential side effects, and ensured he was taking the tablets that needed to accompany the initiation of hormone suppression. At no point did I get any sense that there was a hidden agenda, that there was anything more to the consultation than the task in front of us.

'So I come back for the next one in three months?' he said, tucking his shirt back in afterwards.

He was preparing to leave. I didn't feel I could let him walk out without addressing the issue.

'Yes. And we'll check a blood test then, too.' I hesitated for a second. 'So I remember you coming to see me, to ask about screening, a couple of years ago.'

'That's right.' He had been on his feet, but he sat himself back down beside my desk.

'I wanted to check how you felt about that. Given what's happened. The cancer might have been there then. I didn't know if you wished we'd done your PSA at the time.'

He shook his head briefly. 'I'm not one for looking back. I was glad of all the information you gave me. It made a lot of sense.'

His moustache fanned out slightly when he smiled. 'I'd just retired then. I've had a brilliant time – went all round Canada, and I've played a lot of golf. It's here now and I'll deal with it,' he said. 'Even if it was there back then, I honestly don't think I'd have wanted to know.'

—

At time of writing, Trefor is three years post-diagnosis and remains fit and well, with an undetectable PSA. He attends every three months for ongoing injections, and without fail books those appointments with me. He continues to play an awful lot of golf. I see Michael from time to time about bowel symptoms that, interestingly, echo those of his youngest daughter. He takes no medication, has no sign of heart disease, and has trimmed his weight by means that don't involve the donning of trainers.

Preventative medicine is akin to working one's way along a tightrope, with a plunge into a ravine if balance is lost. Secondary prevention – trying to stop more bad stuff happening to guitar-playing Simon – is uncontroversial. He's actually developed a disease. (The same is true of Anne with her osteoporotic fracture, of course. Even secondary prevention must be considered holistically.) But the whole edifice of primary prevention has very shallow foundations.

Whether it's predicting future ill-health in someone like Michael, or warding off complications in someone like Marta, our 'evidence' is both incomplete and biased towards pharmaceutical interventions. We dress up our risk prediction tools and preventative 'treatments' in the garbs of science, but the emperor is wearing distinctly flimsy clothes. Biomedicine's dirty little secret is how little high-quality evidence we actually have. Even landmark trials such as the UK Prospective Diabetes Study – upon which an entire multimillion-pound industry devoted to the tight control of HbA1c levels has been constructed – has, over the years since publication, attracted ever greater criticism of its substantial flaws. The pressure for academics to demonstrate 'impact' from their research, the financial and lobbying clout of the pharmaceutical industry, the desire among politicians for simple technical fixes to complex socioeconomic issues – all these conspire to drive evermore low- or no-value activity in the NHS. Even the quest to detect cancers through screening presents problems of overdiagnosis and overtreatment that our current level of knowledge ill-equips us to manage. Lives may be saved, but others will be blighted in the process.

The remedy to these quandaries lies in informed consent. How many people today are taking drugs, all of which have the potential to cause harm, with a misplaced faith in their efficacy? What other more holistic opportunities for health promotion are being lost as a result? How many are undergoing tests and procedures the benefits and risks of which are far more nuanced than they imagine? Practitioners with the knowledge, insight, time and skill to navigate the dilemmas are currently the exception rather than the rule.

And by loading responsibility for prevention onto the NHS, our political leaders, swayed by the culture of corporate lobbying, have abdicated their responsibility for the public health. Of course the health service has an important role in disease prevention. But how successful would we have been a generation ago when setting out to tackle tobacco, were our efforts to have been solely confined to the consulting room?

Part Two

TWENTY-FIRST-CENTURY PATIENTS

5

MARTINI MEDICINE

The ringtone woke me at 4 a.m. The chunky Nokia warbling on my bedside table, with its individually illuminated keys and stubby external aerial, belonged to the Oxford practice where I worked. Personal mobile ownership was becoming much more common in the late 1990s but it was still far from ubiquitous. The practice handset with its BT Cellnet contract was passed to whichever doctor was on duty each night or weekend.

'Hello, it's Dr Whitaker.' My words were thick with interrupted sleep.

'Oh, Dr Whitaker, thank you, it's Evelyn Knight.' The voice at the other end spoke quickly. 'It's my husband – he's got this terrible pain in his chest. And he's just been sick.'

I swapped the phone to my other ear and swung my legs out so I was sitting on the side of the bed. My eyes squinted as I switched on the lamp.

'Can I take his name, date of birth, the address and phone number?'

As I spoke, I clicked my pen and straightened the notepad, then took down the details.

'OK, Mrs Knight, thanks. Now, when did this pain come on?'

I ran through a swift history. Yes, it was in the centre of his chest. No, it didn't go anywhere else. Yes, he did look very pale, now I mentioned it. And his breathing was rather heavy.

'I'll be with you very soon, Mrs Knight, but when we put the phone down I want you to ring 999. Your husband may well be having a heart attack. Can you do that?'

There was a catch in her voice when she replied that she would. I told her I was on my way.

I always slept in clothes when I was on call – it was one less thing to do either side of going out, the dressing and undressing. I pulled a jumper over my T-shirt, grabbed my glasses from the desk, and set off through the silent house. I used the spare room when on duty so no one else need be disturbed.

The Abingdon Road, which in a few hours' time would be clogged with commuter traffic, was deserted. I powered my Peugeot 205 south, heading away from the city centre. For less urgent calls I would usually pop into the practice and pick up the patient's Lloyd George envelope, but time was of the essence. There wasn't going to be anything relevant in Gordon Knight's records that I couldn't find out by asking, and I could write my notes up later, after I'd sorted him out.

As I sped along, I thought ahead to what I might find. If this did prove to be a heart attack then things could get very tricky. Oxygen-starved cardiac muscle can at any moment lurch into a chaotic rhythm that no longer provides effective circulation – a cardiac arrest. I could be left trying to resuscitate him on my own on a box-sprung mattress in a cluttered bedroom in the Knights' Cowley home. I imagined the ambulance coursing down Headington Hill, blue lights strafing the trees and houses. Which of us would get there first? My medical bag was in the boot: syringes and needles, diamorphine to bring rapid relief of pain, antiemetic injections to counter nausea, GTN spray to open up blood vessels, aspirin to limit the size of any clot, ampoules of diuretic to drive off fluid backlogging on the lungs. I had everything I needed drugs-wise, and a basic Guedel airway in case of needing to commence CPR. But if things were to go badly, I would really welcome being just one part of a team alongside experienced paramedics.

I'd been in a deep sleep just minutes before, but adrenaline now gave my thoughts a crystal clarity. I reached the junction with Donnington Bridge Road. The traffic lights changed to green as I approached, as though ushering me through. I turned left, accelerating again and crossing the Thames to enter the east of the slumbering city. Evelyn's voice played in my mind: her anxiety, the sudden choking as my words had confirmed her fears. I felt a familiar mixture of exhilaration and sober anticipation, responding to a crisis while the world around me slept.

The Knights' house was the only one with lights on in the street. There was no sign of the ambulance. I retrieved my bag from the boot of the car and within seconds Evelyn was opening the front door to me, her other hand holding her pale green dressing gown closed. Gordon was in bed but conscious and breathing. One look at him, and a hand on his cold clammy skin, told me what I needed to know. I started drawing up my drugs even as I corroborated the history his wife had given on the phone.

The pain of a heart attack can be severe, but more than

that, it is typically accompanied by a deep dread, described as a sense of impending doom. I sited an IV line while Evelyn fetched a glass of water to dissolve the aspirin in. I'd managed dozens of cases during my junior doctor days, and it is one of the most satisfying experiences watching intravenous diamorphine hitting home. Gordon's features, which had been etched with apprehension, softened visibly as his pain dissolved. His arms, which had been pressed to his chest, let go. Evelyn was standing behind me, watching. The tension that charged the air palpably eased a notch or two.

The ambulance arrived. The crew, in green jumpsuits and exuding calm confidence, lugged their kit inside and took my handover. Strapping Gordon into a carry-chair they cracked jokes about who was going to draw the short straw and go first down the Victorian terrace's narrow stairs. I wrote a hasty referral letter on practice notepaper to go with them to the John Radcliffe Hospital. I sat in my car once the blue lights had receded and phoned ahead to the medics to let them know. Gordon's pain had come on less than two hours previously. The hospital team would be ready to get him started on an infusion of a clot-busting drug similar to streptokinase as swiftly as possible – the shorter the 'door to needle time' the more heart muscle would potentially be salvaged, and the better Gordon would ultimately do.

—

That case was more than twenty years ago, yet I remember the details clearly, as I do for several other patients I attended on call as a young GP in Oxford. Some cases were more traumatic. The husband, catching me right at the tail-end of a broken duty night, his wife, terminally ill with metastatic ovarian cancer, crying in the background from sudden, agonising abdominal pain that reflected, I was sure, the erosion of a major blood vessel by tumour. I abandoned breakfast and was there in under ten minutes, and was able to make her final hours pain-free and peaceful. Others were stressful: the feverish, delirious student whose boyfriend phoned when I was tied up with a young woman with a ruptured ectopic pregnancy. Had I been able to get to her, I might have recognised the meningococcal meningitis and given her vital penicillin well before she made it to hospital (thankfully she ultimately fared well).

Most cases, though, have long since faded and are just jumbled, vague memories. Always, though, they were patients of my practice: even if they didn't know me personally they would know my name and that I was part of their team. I could access their records when needed. I would open up the surgery of an evening or over the weekend if it was better to treat them there. And a large percentage of calls didn't need dealing with immediately, many patients' anxieties could be assuaged by advice on the phone or by arranging an appointment for the following day.

There were frustrations. Being woken in the early hours by someone requesting something to help them sleep. Another young man rousing me at midnight to tell me he'd just finished eating some chicken and had realised it was past its date. He was nonplussed to learn he was in the lap of the gods, that there was nothing, right then, that I could do. We had a large, multigenerational Pakistani family on the list who rang, with metronomic regularity, twenty minutes after the surgery had closed. Often there would be several members wanting attention for various non-urgent things. Charitably, the timing might have reflected the father arriving home from work to be confronted by a clutch of problems. But the longer it went on the more obvious it was that they'd worked out a convenient way of bypassing the appointment system. Even frustrations, though, would sometimes pay dividends. Having seen the whole family so often with minor ailments it was instantly obvious when the father was actually unwell. I admitted him that evening with fulminant TB contracted on his recent Hajj.

The level of personal knowledge made for extremely efficient and cost-effective care, and we only troubled the hospital when absolutely necessary. I would know which acute asthmatics could be managed at home and could arrange close follow-up to ensure it had proved safe to do so. A family would be more confident in propping up care for an elderly grandparent, off legs and confused, with a urinary or chest infection, if they knew I would keep the situation under personal review throughout the weekend. But the benefits to the wider NHS, and to our patients of being treated by familiar physicians, was taking an ever-increasing toll. It's one thing to work a full day after a night of broken sleep, or to run through a twelve-day stint with no weekend off in the middle. But to do that month after month, year after year, was becoming untenable. My joining the practice as the fifth pair of hands had come about in an attempt to lighten the load. Neither of the two most senior partners, both in their fifties, could sustain a 1 in 4 rota any longer.

GPs had been covering their own patients round the clock since before the advent of the NHS, but around us the world was changing. Sunday trading, later licensing hours: the 24/7 society was gathering pace. Other sectors such as banking and insurance were extending hours into evenings and weekends, and using first telephone then the internet instead of physical high-street branches. Convenience for consumers, efficiency for employers: powerful forces increasingly pushed demand for services outside traditional working hours. Medical care was no exception. The distinction between urgent and routine matters was becoming progressively blurred – we were entering the era of Martini medicine: any time, any place, anywhere. Additionally, the growing fashion for awareness-raising campaigns – Could it be meningitis? – heightened anxiety and lowered many people's thresholds for seeking advice at the first hint of trouble.

We were the last practice in the city still to do our own on-call. Most surgeries had already opted for one of two alternative solutions to the ever-rising workload of GP out-of-hours. The more popular was membership of the GP cooperative: multiple practices joining forces to provide cover on a rota basis, sharing the burden of disrupted sleep and lost weekends among a large pool of doctors. Shifts were non-stop – calls would come in from patients from all participating surgeries – but each individual GP was rostered to be on duty far less frequently. It was possible to arrange time off following a duty period to allow for recovery. And the remainder of the evenings, nights and weekends were free for family life, leisure interests and the recharging of batteries. Although patients would now most often be seen by a doctor from a surgery other than their own, the care remained of a high standard. The doctors in the area all knew one another, if not personally then certainly by reputation. No one would want to become known among their peers as being a buck-passer or for taking shortcuts with people's care.

A few practices preferred to subcontract some or all of their out-of-hours duties to commercial deputising services, paying money to be liberated from having to participate in any rota at all. There were many good locums working for such organisations, but by no means all were. And there were few if any personal links between them and the GP partners whose patients they were caring for. Agency doctors, often drafted in from elsewhere – even flying in from abroad, and wholly unfamiliar with the NHS and with local services – were employed to fill rota gaps. Run on tight economic lines, ratios of GPs to workload were poor. Under-referral and over-referral to hospital – each bad for different reasons – were far from rare, the harried, often junior and relatively inexperienced deputising doctors having little time or incentive to engage with anything complex or involved.

Even those practices using commercial services still retained twenty-four-hour responsibility for their patients. There would always have to be a nominated partner available to step in at no notice should the deputising service be unable to supply cover, either because of staff shortages or sickness, or overwhelming workload. All GPs had endured punishing hours during their years of training spent as junior doctors, but legal challenges and sustained political pressure were now leading to steady improvements in conditions for our hospital colleagues. General practice, with its unlimited responsibility for patient care, was an increasingly unattractive career option. In 2002, the oldest partner in our practice retired. Despite national advertising, we were unable to recruit a suitable replacement. What had once been a highly desirable proposition – a partnership in a prestigious practice in the heart of a beautiful university city – was no longer something the new generation seemed to want to do.

—

Twenty-odd years later, 2021. Nine-year-old Ryan's case was highlighted in red on the triage screen, demanding an urgent callback. NHS Pathways, the algorithmic software used by NHS 111, had deemed that an emergency ambulance should be dispatched.

I got through to his father, Tony. 'It's Dr Whitaker from the out-of-hours GP service,' I explained. 'I gather you called 111 about your son – I'm ringing to see how best to help. What's been going on?'

'Not a lot really.' Tony sounded bemused. 'He was sick on the bus home from school.'

I ran through a checklist. Did he have a fever, rash or headache? Was light troubling him? Did he strike his father as confused? 'No, honestly, he's fine,' Tony assured me. 'He only chucked up the once. I put it down to travel sickness.'

It was now 7.30 in the evening. Ryan had eaten a normal dinner. 'What made you phone 111 then?' I asked.

Tony explained that kids with vomiting or diarrhoea were supposed to stay off school until they'd been symptom-free for forty-eight hours. Given that he felt Ryan's nausea was travel-related rather than due to a tummy bug, he'd rung the school to ask whether it would be OK to send him in the following day. They'd told him to give 111 a call and take their advice. Not being the slightest bit concerned about his son's condition, he'd sorted out the evening meal first. It had been a complete surprise when, rather than answer his query, the 111 call handler had told him they were sending an ambulance straight away.

These scenarios are incredibly common. I encounter them numerous times in every out-of-hours shift. The call-handlers are not clinicians. Their role is to plug the details of each case into NHS Pathways and follow its recommended action. And Pathways doesn't generate advice. It simply seeks to determine what kind of service the patient should access and how quickly. Pathways is also highly risk-averse. Pretty much any symptom you can think of might just be indicative of an urgent problem. In around 20% of all calls handled by 111, Pathways recommends ambulances be dispatched or patients should attend A&E, yet in the vast majority the problem is far from serious – Ryan's details had triggered just such an overreaction. In an attempt to stem the flood of these inappropriate outcomes, the GP out-of-hours service in our area now tries to intercept as many of them as it can. I told Tony that the ambulance would be stood down, and as long as Ryan remained well he could attend school in the morning.

If a GP could get to every one of these erroneous Pathways dispositions in time, my experience suggests we would divert 90% of the unnecessary A&E attendances and ambulance call-outs generated by 111. Put another way, for every 100 NHS 111 calls, Pathways sends twenty into the emergency services, whereas a GP would send just two. Yet there are far too few doctors to enable this. The large commercial organisation that I now undertake out-of-hours work for struggles perennially to fill its rota. That picture is true nationwide, with services frequently staffed with fewer than half the required numbers of GPs. (I've chosen not to clutter this book with too many figures, but it's worth noting that – according to health think tank The King's Fund – it costs the NHS £36 if a GP like me deals with one of these cases, over £200 if an ambulance is dispatched, and if the patient is taken needlessly to hospital then the bill is anywhere north of £400.)

The dwindling pool of doctors still undertaking out-of-hours duties is simultaneously left trying to manage a hugely expanded workload. Over a typical weekend, the triage screen will swell unmanageably, often as many as 300 cases awaiting a callback from a clinician. Partly this is because NHS 111 has been sold to the public as a source of medical advice 24/7 when in fact it is merely a risk-averse triaging service, so time and again people like Tony find themselves unwittingly sucked into the urgent-care system. Then there is the related crisis in daytime general practice. The total GP workforce has been declining steadily since 2015 and in under-doctored areas practices no longer have sufficient capacity to meet their patients' in-hours needs. The default when all appointments have gone – as frequently happens within half an hour of the phone lines opening – is to direct callers to NHS 111. This sets up circles of frustration and despair for patients. For anyone with a problem requiring non-urgent GP care – whether that's correctly recognised by Pathways or whether they're sent instead into A&E, the ambulance service, or GP out-of-hours – the ultimate outcome for many is simply to be told to go back to their overwhelmed surgery and try again.

As little as five years ago it was a rarity for me to speak to paramedics. Now I do so multiple times every shift. NHS 111 ambulance dispatches that haven't been intercepted frequently result in paramedics tied up with patients who don't require their skills. We try to get back to them as quickly as possible so as to formulate an appropriate management plan, and liberate them to get back out on the road for genuine emergencies again.

—

I arranged to meet Andrew Wilson (his name has been changed) for a pint at The Globe at Newton St Loe. Although we work alongside each other these days at the out-of-hours service, there's never time for more than friendly greetings. And I was especially interested in Andrew's experiences because, commencing as it did in 2004, his ambulance service career spanned exactly the era I wanted better to understand.

After sixteen years of working for an office equipment repair company, Andrew was looking for a new challenge. He initially decided to swap defunct franking machines for an L-plated dual-control car. He'd got two-thirds of the way to qualifying as a driving instructor when he chanced upon an advert recruiting prospective ambulance technicians to work in the high-dependency unit with the local ambulance service.

The job, when he looked into it, greatly appealed: he'd be able to make a real difference to people in need. The HDU primarily focused on 'Paeds Retrievals' – transferring critically ill children to the appropriate specialist centres – and

'Doctors Urgents' – patients like Gordon Knight who'd been assessed by a GP as needing immediate conveyance for hospital care. The prospect threw him into indecision; no longer did driving instruction seem the path to pursue. He decided to apply. And the ambulance service seemed delighted to have him.

'The first five, six years it was a "proper" ambulance job,' he told me. 'We'd be going to heart attacks, acute asthma, major trauma. There were road traffic collisions that were quite horrific.'

The gravity of the call-outs might deter some, but Andrew thrived in his new role. Outside his former day job he'd had years of experience as a captain with the army reserves, teaching survival skills and orienteering during exacting training expeditions on Dartmoor. Calmness and leadership under pressure were in his blood. And it was an exciting era in which to be in the ambulance service. The first pilot projects training ambulance drivers beyond basic first aid began in the 1970s. In recognition that they would frequently be first attenders in cases of significant injury or illness, skills had been progressively enhanced over the ensuing decades, leading to the evolution of an entirely new role, that of paramedic, able to administer a range of emergency drugs and perform advanced life support. When Andrew joined the service, the role was extending even further. Evidence was accumulating that the earlier clot-busting drugs could be given to heart attack victims, the better their outcomes. To circumvent the delays arising from transportation, especially in rural areas, in the early 2000s paramedics began to administer thrombolytic injections to confirmed heart attack victims before taking them into A&E.

This new discipline, becoming known as pre-hospital emergency medicine (PHEM), demanded ever greater education and competencies. From 2007, training for new paramedics became university-based. Seeing his ambulance technician role being downgraded and keen to develop further, Andrew enrolled on a four-year programme with the Open University, studying alongside his full-time job. In 2013 he qualified as a fully-fledged paramedic.

Yet while Andrew was riding this wave towards ever greater scope and responsibility in the provision of out-of-hospital emergency care, other changes were occurring. In 2010, the government launched the new non-emergency number, NHS 111.

'In Avon,' he said, referring to the name his ambulance service had at the time, 'we'd get between six and seven hundred calls a night – that would go up to twelve hundred on New Year's Eve. When they introduced 111, it instantly doubled the numbers. It turned every night into a New Year's Eve.'

These additional cases were of a different type, patients whose queries triggered the risk-averse Pathways software inappropriately. Used to attending asthmatics in extremis, Andrew recalls being blue-lighted to a patient who had simply misplaced his inhaler. The man had been apologetic: 'I told 111 this but they said they had to send someone to check me over.' Sometimes a whole shift would be spent with Andrew attending low acuity calls that simply didn't require his training and expertise. And it was a service-wide problem. In his clinical team-leader role, Andrew had management oversight of call volumes and case mix. 'It was astounding the number and trivial things that 111 put through.' The problem can't be solved simply by adjusting the Pathways algorithms. As we'll see in the next chapter, no AI can accurately diagnose and manage risk like a human clinician. In order to be safe, Pathways and its non-clinical call-handlers must overreact in a substantial proportion of cases.

It has led to a whole new category of paramedic outcome: leave at home. 'It used to be that, nine out of ten times, you'd give the drugs you had then take the patient to hospital.' Now Andrew was being called to numerous patients with non-urgent problems who manifestly didn't require paramedic or hospital care, yet he still had to go through everything in the same immense level of detail. The service, he explained, was unforgiving if decisions ever proved to have been flawed. 'Every call takes between an hour and an hour and twenty minutes. You've got to get everything perfect. If something goes wrong, you're the first to be held up for blame.'

Some patients with obviously minor issues – green category – he would decide autonomously to leave at home. But many would be amber – not requiring admission, but with complex or undifferentiated problems that needed GP input to devise a safe management plan. It could add at least thirty minutes to a case just waiting for a doctor to call back and talk the uncertainties through. Paramedics, highly skilled at responding to emergency situations, were being expected to deal time and again with patients their training, processes and procedures had never been prepared for.

'It grinds you down, you get angry. You think: why is this still happening? Why are we being asked to do this?'

This radical alteration of case mix and role – completely

mismatched to traditional paramedic skills and motivation – has caused widespread disenchantment. Some have responded by super-specialisation, undertaking further training to be able to secure a scarce place on dedicated trauma teams that deal only with high-acuity incidents. Those that are left within the general service face a job radically different from that for which they trained, and many vote with their feet. 'When I joined,' Andrew said, 'paramedics left the service in two ways: retired, or in a box.' In one month alone, recently, he recalls twenty resigning from just two stations in the area.

To try to plug the gaps, the NHS is recruiting heavily from abroad – something I've noticed myself, speaking to increasing numbers of paramedics with South African, Polish or Antipodean accents. 'They come from countries where they're doing what we used to do,' Andrew explained. 'They've got no idea about the NHS and the culture they're joining.' They often don't last long. He is scathing about the response to the unprecedented levels of staff turnover. 'It's like a World War One situation, just throwing more and more troops over the top, instead of dealing with the source of the problem.'

—

Back in 2002, faced with a retiring senior partner and with no suitable recruit to replace him, my Oxford practice had to make do with what we could find. An established GP, leaving a partnership in a different county, seemed to have coherent motivations: a desire to move his family for quality of life and educational opportunities. The logistics of these things can be difficult: children should ideally relocate at the end of a school year, and then there's the business of finding a new home. But after six months of him commuting for hours each day, and sleeping on a camp bed in surgery when on call, it became apparent that whatever might be going on in his life, it wasn't a desired family move.

After he left, a doctor from a nearby surgery in the city got in touch. He'd heard we were finding it hard to fill our vacancy. He would be interested. His reasons for leaving his current practice seemed plausible enough; he and his partners had apparently fallen out. And that could have accounted for his inability to produce references from current colleagues. We had niggling reservations but he was someone we knew from round and about. And we were by then in the position of beggars, not choosers. The honeymoon lasted a little while but cracks started to show: late to start surgeries, days off unwell. One afternoon he appeared to have vanished from the building and after an extensive search he was found slumped in the loo, comatose from the drug he had tragically become addicted to.

Our recruitment challenges were being replicated around the country. Something had to be done to make general practice an attractive career again. The answer was an entirely new contract, agreed with the profession in 2004. This was the contract that introduced QOF, bringing with it a significant boost to practice funding. The other key feature was liberation from twenty-four-hour responsibility. GPs would still provide all care for patients during the core hours of 8 a.m. to 6.30 p.m. But in return for losing the income derived from performing night visits, the onerous task of covering evenings and weekends was to be passed to the bodies that ran the NHS in each locality, primary care trusts (PCTs).

The 2004 contract achieved its aims. With its QOF-derived boost to remuneration, and the end of twenty-four-hour responsibility, younger doctors wanted to become GPs again. Recruitment surged, and posts of a new type, enabled by another change in the contract, became commonplace: that of a salaried GP, employed by a partnership to undertake purely clinical work, but with no responsibility or risk for owning and running the practice. Earnings, though, were commensurately lower and there was soon a growing clamour from salaried doctors frustrated at the lack of available partnership posts. Just a few years after a new contract had dramatically improved terms and conditions, practices like mine in Oxford, formerly unable to replace a retiring partner, were being inundated by applications whenever a vacancy arose.

I myself had relocated by then and have watched from the vantage of my long-term partnership near Bath as the once hailed 2004 contract has been slowly revealed as a poisoned chalice. The effects of QOF on medical practice are dealt with elsewhere in the book, here I will focus on the chaos and deterioration the 2004 contract has caused in the provision of urgent medical care when surgery doors are closed.

Initially, no one would have noticed any change. PCTs had absolutely no experience of providing the out-of-hours services that had suddenly been landed in their laps, so most subcontracted the task straight back to the established GP cooperatives to organise. But now, working out of hours was something doctors could choose, rather than be obliged to do. And people did. Lots of us – to start with. Shifts were so popular that our co-op had to limit each doctor to a maximum of five per month in order to ensure everyone had a fair share. What had turned this previously burdensome aspect of GP life into such an attractive proposition? The elements of choice and control were undoubtedly important, but the key factor was remuneration. Prior to the 2004 contract, GPs were compelled to provide evening, night, weekend and public holiday cover for their patients 365 days of the year for a sum that averaged out at £10 per hour. At a stroke, that rate was increased eightfold. Suddenly, out-of-hours work was something for which enthusiasm was breathtakingly renewed.

The dearth of GPs undertaking out-of-hours work these days is a direct result of a gradual reversal of that process. As the decade of austerity ground on, the NHS was subjected to the most sustained real-terms funding squeeze in its history. PCTs, and their 2013 replacements, clinical commissioning groups (CCGs), sought economies wherever they could. And the bill for providing out-of-hours services seemed a low-hanging fruit. Terms and conditions for GPs have been progressively eroded. I continue to undertake a shift each week – for me it is part of the role of a doctor, responding to the crises and concerns that strike when routine services have gone home, and I enjoy the variety and acuity of the cases. Yet my pay for performing exactly the same work is 20% lower than it was sixteen years ago – and that's not taking any account of the impact of inflation over the intervening years. Little wonder that so many of my colleagues have decided that sacrificing evening, night or weekend time is no longer for them. The retreat of experienced clinicians from the out-of-hours environment, and the attempt to replace them with a computer-based service – superficially cheaper, but which leads to huge costs and consequences in the emergency services – has been a disastrous political miscalculation.

—

Andrew resigned from the ambulance service in 2020 and took up a post within our out-of-hours organisation as a clinical responder. It was a brand-new role intended to be filled by paramedics, which has arisen in response to the dearth of GPs. He and his growing band of colleagues spend their shifts doing home visits to all except very young children and patients needing end-of-life care.

In that respect, he's dealing with just the sort of amber cases that have come to swamp the ambulance service, yet now he enjoys the work. Rather than fearing criticism and blame should a decision about a complex or uncertain situation prove to have been wrong, he feels well supported. Assessment procedures are designed specifically for the type of patients he sees, and he and his fellow clinical responders have a dedicated GP on the phone with whom they discuss all cases once seen.

I wondered if he missed the drama of the high-acuity call-outs for which he had undergone his extensive paramedic training. He greeted the question with a wry smile. 'I still do occasional bank shifts for the ambulance service,' he said, 'and I dread going in for them.' Initially he was tempted to put it down to being fifty-two: 'Perhaps at my age I no longer need the adrenaline.' But as we talked further, it seemed the explanations were more complicated. In the early years of his career, the vast majority of his call-outs were to genuine emergencies, and despite the high stakes there is something psychologically helpful about consistency. If you know that every case you're attending is likely to need the full deployment of your training then you're always prepared. It's altogether more unnerving to be blue-lighted to patient after patient, never knowing which out of the slew of undifferentiated and low-grade illness might actually prove to be life-threatening.

There were other themes besides. Low morale permeating the service. Feeling vulnerable to being scapegoated through lack of management support in a radically altered role. The rigidity of pathways and protocols that allow no clinical discretion and insist on laborious processes and procedures in scenarios for which they were never designed.

University paramedic departments are adapting to the new realities, transforming their courses to train new graduates in wide-ranging generalist skills in an attempt to prepare them for the huge range of complexity and variable acuity they're likely to meet, including in mental health (something Andrew never encountered in his early years, yet which is now a frequent part of a paramedic's workload). Time and again one finds reference to biopsychosocial assessment and diagnosis. When I look through these new curricula, it strikes me the training is now attempting to turn the next generation of paramedics into replacements for GPs.

—

The changes I've witnessed in out-of-hours care are beginning to be mirrored in the daytime setting. In my early years of practice, GPs would provide urgent care both out of hours, as I did for Gordon Knight, and also in daytime practice. Patients with pressing problems would be accommodated in various ways – walk-in surgeries, duty doctor sessions, appointments reserved for booking on the day. We never turned them away. At any moment we might have to abandon a clinic and dash out on an urgent home visit. On most occasions these unscheduled cases would prove to be patients we could manage at home, but where they required admission or pre-hospital emergency care, we would be greatly appreciative of the back-up provided by our paramedic colleagues.

The post-2004 contract recruitment boom is well and truly over: the number of whole-time equivalent GPs has been falling steadily for years. We now have nearly 10% fewer than in 2015, while the patient population continues to increase in both size and complexity. This new crisis in recruitment and retention, coupled with the anxieties and expectations among patients for near instant access, has left under-doctored practices seeking to plug gaps in service provision with other professionals. Home visits are a time-consuming part of a GP's day, traffic and travel distances often chewing up hours. Many areas have launched home visiting services, staffed by paramedics like Andrew disillusioned with the ambulance service. And increasingly, surgeries unable to meet the demand for same-day appointments are looking to locally based urgent-care hubs as the solution to relieve the pressures they're under.

I have the greatest respect for my colleagues in allied professions. Were I to suffer a heart attack, or a head injury, or be involved in a serious road traffic accident, it is paramedics I would want on scene – and absolutely not a GP like me. But our skill sets are completely different. It takes a minimum of ten years before a doctor is licensed to practise independently as a GP, and the breadth and depth of our training and experience equips us to manage complex or uncertain scenarios swiftly, safely, efficiently and holistically. The gradual retreat of the declining GP workforce from providing daytime urgent care will create the same fragmentation and inefficiencies that have come to blight services out of hours – and will have the same deleterious consequences for the emergency services. And it is leading to a near absence of GP care for many of our most vulnerable patients – be they the frail multimorbid housebound elderly who rely on home visits to see their doctor, anxious individuals presenting with serial seemingly unconnected complaints, or chaotic families in desperate need of biopsychosocial care.

The changes Andrew has lived through are an inverted image of those in my own career.

Perhaps the greatest lesson to be learned is their completely unplanned nature. How bold policy responses like the 2004 GP contract cause enduring consequences that are as unintended as they were unforeseen. Likewise the advent of NHS 111, flooding patient groups into parts of the system not geared to deal with their problems. How erosions in terms and conditions for healthcare professionals have set off chain reactions with which the NHS is still grappling and trying to work out its response. Caught up in this ongoing tumult are patients, unwell and worried, too often failing to get the care they need in a timely manner from an

NHS struggling to adapt post-hoc and piecemeal to the fallout from policy decisions that were launched but never properly managed.

It's a theme we will return to elsewhere in this book. Meanwhile, Andrew and I sat finishing our drinks in The Globe, paramedic and doctor, neither of us entirely certain what it is these days that we are actually supposed to be.

6

DOCTOR GOOGLE AND THE AI REVOLUTION

Gary was unshaven and restless. He kept pressing his hands to different places on his chest as he tried to describe the pain he'd been experiencing, and the difficulty breathing, and the sick feeling and light-headedness. At twenty-two, these were unlikely to represent a serious heart or lung problem – unlikely, though by no means impossible. But I'd skimmed his notes before calling him through to my consulting room. They were the same symptoms he'd been experiencing a year or so previously. He'd been extensively investigated and nothing worrying had been found. The last time I'd seen him, I'd tried to broker the understanding that they must represent physical manifestations of anxiety. I'd started him on some medication and arranged to see him a few weeks later, hoping that if he were responding it would increase his confidence in my diagnosis. He hadn't returned.

Lola, his girlfriend, sitting in the other chair, was hostile. 'He keeps getting fobbed off, being told there's nothing wrong.' Gary's notes contained records of multiple 111 contacts. As soon as he mentioned chest pain and breathing difficulties to the operator, high drama would ensue. A paramedic ambulance would be dispatched. Which would rush him, blue lights flashing, to the nearest A&E. Where doctors clad in scrubs would do all manner of tests, after which he'd be told they were normal and he'd be sent home.

'I'm not fobbing you off,' I told them. 'There's definitely something wrong, and I really want to help. But I need you to work with me.'

I started to explain why, if he kept phoning 111, he was likely to remain stuck in the same unproductive loop.

'I know the symptoms are really unpleasant,' I said. 'I guess at times it must feel like you're about to collapse.'

Gary nodded, his lips pressing together.

'But I can absolutely assure you: you're not going to. There's no sign of anything like that.'

This provoked a dismissive huff from Lola. 'You're saying it's all in his head.'

'You're not imagining it,' I said to him. 'The symptoms are real, and they feel horrible. But I do think they're caused by stress. Some people experience anxiety in their minds, but for others it comes out in the body. All that adrenaline pumping round – it causes symptoms just like you get.'

'Those tablets didn't work, though,' Gary pointed out.

'They take a little while,' I said. 'You never gave them long enough.'

We talked briefly through what was going on in his life. Gary had wanted to trace his biological father, from whom he hadn't heard since he was a kid. It had caused huge ructions with his mum and step-dad the previous year and all the turmoil had proved to have been pointless. When

Gary finally tracked him down he was too late, his biological dad had died some six months before. Now Lola was pregnant with their first and Gary was facing the prospect of becoming a father to a little one of his own. I was sure his physical symptoms reflected repressed grief and abandonment being mightily stirred.

There was zero appetite for psychological therapy. In the end, they left with a prescription for another medication and agreed to return in three weeks. I wondered whether they would. Everything they read online – googling 'chest pain' and 'difficulty breathing' – told them there must be something serious going on. And that belief was reinforced by the dramatic response to his 111 calls – sirens, monitors, blood tests and ECGs – albeit that nothing ever seemed to come of it. There was such a contrast between those experiences and my low-key attribution of his symptoms to psychological ill-health. The confusion that Gary and Lola must feel. Who were they to trust? What if it was a heart problem, a lung pathology, and nobody had put their finger on it yet? The papers were always screaming about how flawed the medical profession can be – *Four doctors missed meningitis! GPs failing to spot cancer!* I must look like the next bungling idiot about to generate another set of scornful headlines. Little wonder it was so hard for them to know what to believe.

—

Even though we'd started Harriet on twenty-minute appointments, with strategic gaps to allow her to make up time, her surgery had run very late. When she finally got to the end,

I went through to debrief. There were bits of paper strewn across her desk, reminding her to do tasks that she hadn't had time for during the consultations themselves. She had not one but two stethoscopes draped around her neck, where she'd hurriedly parked them after conducting examinations. Her eyes had a startled distraction to them, as though she was still trying to work out what had just hit her. I pulled up a chair and gave her a smile.

'Don't worry. How you're feeling is entirely normal.'

We started to go through her cases. She'd got bogged down by a middle-aged woman with abdominal pain, fatigue and irregular vaginal bleeding. An older chap on multiple medications for heart disease, emphysema, diabetes, prostate problems and blood pressure who was feeling unsteady and muzzy-headed and forgetful. A child who for months now had been making bizarre facial grimaces at random times and who was falling behind at school. Someone else with chronic pain in their muscles and joints with a normal set of investigations.

I talked her through each case, encouraging her whenever I felt she'd come up with a good plan, and gently expanding on other things to think about or alternative approaches she could have taken when a patient's presentation had left her perplexed.

'I just feel so pathetic,' she said when we finally finished.

I told her I'd felt exactly the same at her stage, and that everyone else does, too. GP registrars study and train for a minimum of nine years – virtually all of them spent in the hospital environment – before setting foot in primary care. Nothing prepares them for their first weeks. The 'medical model' – which essentially views a human being as a complex machine that can go wrong in numerous but always eminently explicable ways – works well in hospitals. Those are the kinds of patients one usually encounters there, people with 'organic' pathology – diseases with abnormalities identifiable on blood tests, X-rays, scans, biopsies and the like. But out in general practice the medical model falls apart spectacularly. Yes, some of the time we do see patients with barn-door organic problems and then it's usually reasonably straightforward to know what to do. It's all the others – the people with bewildering combinations of complaints that don't fit with what one finds in textbooks, others whose apparently textbook cases turn out to be anything but – those make up the majority of our work. Appointment after appointment we are presented with undifferentiated symptomatology – tired all the time, chronic cough, mysterious headaches, bowels gone haywire. We have to be careful not to miss anything important. At the same time we have to learn new ways to make sense of it all.

I outlined for Harriet the bare bones of the biopsychosocial model, which all GPs become adept at using over time. How the 'bio' bit – the medical model – is only one part of the picture. When a patient like Gary comes to see her she'll be perfectly capable of seeking out organic causes: heart problems, asthma, blood clots on the lungs. But in his case, she would draw a blank. The task for her now was to build an understanding of how people's emotions, psychology, personality, family, relationships, occupation, material circumstances, lifestyle, experiences, hopes and fears all interact with their biology in a glorious mishmash to create the kinds of stories they come to tell us. It's the arena in which medicine is powerfully revealed to be not just a science, nor even an art. It's where medicine is most properly understood to be a humanity.

'Give it six, eight weeks,' I told her. 'You'll start to get the hang of it.'

—

When I was growing up in the 1970s and 80s, my parents had a copy of *The Home Doctor* on their bookshelf. It was an A–Z guide to 150 common conditions, with advice on self-care remedies and first aid treatments. My dad wrote the dates on which my brother, sister and I had contracted the common childhood illnesses – chickenpox, mumps and so on – on the inside front cover, so he'd know once we'd got past them all. I've no idea whether he used the same book to look up scrotal lumps when he noticed the swelling in his testicle. Whether he'd sat tight, stewing – trying to persuade himself, hope against hope, that what he'd found might be the result of one of the harmless potential causes listed there: a cyst, a hernia, a knot of varicose veins – before finally deciding he needed to make an appointment with our family GP, Dr Forshaw.

Books like *The Home Doctor* – augmented by articles in glossy women's magazines and agony aunt columns in the papers – were pretty much the extent of publicly available medical information in that era. Nevertheless, unless they were pressingly severe, people have always sought to make sense of their symptoms before consulting with professionals. As a GP registrar in the mid-1990s I was impressed by research that showed that the typical patient would have polled an average of twelve different sources of information before turning up in surgery. The experiences and opinions of a spouse, parents, siblings, friends, neighbours and work colleagues would very likely have been sought. These networks might have thrown up an example of a cousin, say, who'd had something similar, or an article or programme that someone remembered that seemed to fit the bill. All this information would be weighed and considered as part of the decision as to whether to go to the doctor, and would inform what the patient was concerned must be wrong.

The need to evaluate the meaning of symptoms or bodily changes is a human constant, and since the late 1990s the internet has brought an explosion in the availability of information. Those dozen sources of yesteryear now seem piddling, given the entirety of the medical literature accessible from the smartphone in anyone's pocket. Sites like nhs.uk or patient.info generally supply authoritative information geared to the general public. Raw research papers from numerous scientific journals can be open-accessed. Forums such as Mumsnet enable people to swap experiences from anywhere in the world. And alternative approaches, misinformation and conspiracy theories jostle to make their perspectives known.

This phenomenal wealth of information and interpretation has given rise to a hybrid *Home Doctor* for the digital age, known by patients and physicians alike as Dr Google. Sometimes his/her advice can be bang on. I've occasionally had patients come in with a ready worked out diagnosis that proves to be right. But such instances are rare. Far more common is alarm. There are roughly 200 symptoms a human can experience, yet there are approximately 6,000 diseases (and 4,000 medication side effects). And each disease may present in different ways, depending on the patient. Pretty much any symptom you can think of *might* be an indication of cancer, or multiple sclerosis, or some other pathology that one really wouldn't want to have. When Gary and Lola try typing his chest pain and difficulty breathing into a search box, they're instantly persuaded there must be something serious going on. Dr Google is excellent at generating worst-case scenarios, but appallingly bad at context.

The internet has transformed things for doctors. Once I've got things into the right context – once I've made a diagnosis – I can point people in the direction of reliable web resources. Research shows that patients remember at most three things from a typical consultation. Now I can provide them with links to good quality, relevant information to read and re-read at their own pace in the comfort of home. They can discover things to improve matters for themselves, or different ideas for treatment from that which I might have recommended. Equipped with reliable and appropriate information, patients can become experts in their own health.

From my own perspective, if I want to brush up on the optimum way to manage, say, a flare of inflammatory bowel disease, I no longer need to take a trip to the library to seek out a review article in a medical journal, I can call up the evidence on my desktop there and then. Faced with an unusual scenario – a teenage virgin who's passed a large triangular mass of fleshy tissue during an unusually painful period, say – I can rustle up the answer with a bit of canny searching. In enlisting Dr Google to solve diagnostic puzzles,

I do so having spent decades inhabiting the medical world. I can make a good stab at what search terms to use, which sources can be relied on and which discounted and skipped over, and I can put what I find into the appropriate context for the patient in front of me.

Harriet was still in the earliest phases of her journey. Steeped for years in the medical model in hospital practice, she could use online resources to update her knowledge about organic diseases and to supply patients with information once diagnoses had been securely made. But the painful dislocation she was currently experiencing reflected the challenge ahead, something there was no way to circumvent and for which she would need the guidance of an experienced trainer – the slow, incremental accumulation of new knowledge and experience of the art and the humanity of medicine, things that would in time allow her to function effectively as a fully-fledged GP.

What, though, if Dr Google had the same kind of context-setting skills as a human doctor like me? What if Dr Google, rather than simply chucking out worst-case scenarios, could actually come up with something tailored to the individual seeking help. In short, what if Dr Google could actually make accurate diagnoses?

What might that mean for patients? Convenience – able to find out what was wrong instantaneously? Or shock and anxiety – perhaps scrolling their phone apprehensively late at night, or during their morning commute, only to find bad news?

What might that mean for the NHS, presented with a technological workaround to the expense of training and retaining tens of thousands of GPs?

What might that mean for Harriet? And what might that mean for me?

—

In 2018, I was working an out-of-hours shift alongside Jürgen, a German doctor with an entrepreneurial spirit and an interest in medical technology. He showed me an app on his phone – something called GP at Hand, supplied by a company called Babylon – which Jürgen had downloaded to play with. At the time, Babylon was making controversial inroads into providing general practice services to people in London – controversial because they had very few physical facilities in which to actually see patients. Video consultations were the default for those who were ultimately deemed in need of human attention. Their GP at Hand app was the service's front door.

Jürgen was enthusiastic. 'Look, this is what they use – they don't even need people to see a doctor. You put in your symptom,' he said, swiping and tapping at his screen, 'it goes through some questions and – there! Look, it tells you what's wrong!'

I thought Jürgen was over-excited. What I saw of the app, looking over his shoulder, struck me as rigid and unwieldy – question after question, yes-no, yes-no. The examples he was trialling – straightforward issues like sore throat or new-onset diarrhoea – seemed eventually to result in sensible suggestions, though these were always presented as a list of possibilities rather than a definitive diagnosis, so patients would still be left trying to work out which was the right one. Not much of an advance on Dr Google. And I couldn't see it being of use with the kinds of complex, multifaceted cases I spend much of my days on. I filed it in a mental box marked 'interesting gimmick' and thought no more about it.

A few months later, Babylon was suddenly in the headlines. They claimed they'd pitted GP at Hand against the exam all doctors have to pass before being allowed to practise as GPs – the MRCGP – and it had sailed through with 81%, a higher mark than some of the seven human doctors enlisted by Babylon to sit the same paper. Ali Parsa, Babylon's CEO, was being interviewed in every publication I came across. He described the results as 'phenomenal'. 'You study your whole life to become a GP . . . For a machine to be able to pass this with flying colours in its first go, that is incredible.'

Matt Hancock, then Secretary of State for Health, was seduced, no doubt dazzled by a vision of providing healthcare with a smaller and far less expensive workforce. He shared a platform with Parsa at a presentation from Babylon's HQ extolling the AI revolution, and announced that he wanted GP at Hand rolled out across the entire NHS as a matter of prime importance.

I thought back to Jürgen. Perhaps he'd been right to be so excited about the app, maybe I'd misjudged it. But the thought gave me a feeling of foreboding. I had no idea how Babylon had achieved the incredible performance they claimed. Like many a person in mid-life or beyond confronted by technological wizardry outwith their experience, I felt intimidated. Parsa's explanations simply baffled me:

> The way we train the machine is very novel. No one else in the world is doing it. Our approach of mixing a knowledge

> base with natural language processing, a probabilistic graphical model and inference engine – put on top of a deep learning engine – allowed us to achieve the results at a speed that nobody else could.

I had no idea what he was talking about. I had an overpowering sense that the world was passing me by.

Whatever it was Babylon had been doing, they proved to be far from the only ones. Soon 'symptom checker' apps seemed to be everywhere, multiple competitors crowding the marketplace. The consumer magazine *Which?* ran a feature article comparing their relative performances. The NHS, responding to Hancock's exhortations, seemed to be heading full speed towards adopting these new technologies. Practices were to be compelled to offer patients online access and many of the platforms were aping Babylon's approach and incorporating a symptom checker at the front door. There was fevered talk about apps like this diverting many patients towards self-care, or perhaps advice from a pharmacist, thereby solving the problem of burgeoning workload in general practice. Armed with a reassuring diagnosis from their smartphone, how many people might no longer even feel the need to see their GP?

—

'We started twenty years back. I didn't even know we were doing AI then. It was only three or four years ago when someone said: that's what you're doing.'

It was the following year, 2019, and I was speaking with Jason Maude, co-founder of Isabel Healthcare. The video-conferencing software we were supposed to be using for the call hadn't worked, so we made do with the phone, Maude demonstrating Isabel's functionality on my computer through a screen-sharing mode.

Maude's earlier career was as a financial analyst. But then his three-year-old daughter, Isabel, suffered a potentially fatal complication of chickenpox, which was initially misdiagnosed by the junior doctors looking after her. Isabel survived – just – but spent months in a critical condition in hospital. The disaster arose because her physicians hadn't been aware of the existence of the extremely rare complication she'd developed and had initially misinterpreted her decline in terms of the original viral infection. When Maude came to understand this, he abandoned his former career and set about developing a computer tool to help doctors generate alternative diagnoses in puzzling or unusual clinical scenarios. Isabel Healthcare Ltd was born.

'Computers are pretty dumb,' Maude explained, 'but they're very good at doing a very narrow job.' The Isabel engine works a bit like a highly specialised Google search. Its database is fed huge quantities of medical literature – textbooks, journals, case reports – building up comprehensive pictures of the entire range of symptoms and signs associated with virtually any known medical condition. A user can enter a free-text description of their case, Isabel will interpret it and churn through its database of some 6,000 diseases and 4,000 drug side effects to find matches for the pattern. The list of potential diagnoses is then ranked by relevance or how well they fit. For much of Isabel's existence her users have been doctors – she was originally designed as a tool for physicians, to help them generate and consider alternative causes when they had any doubt as to what might be wrong. Latterly, since it was pointed out to Maude that what he was doing was AI, Isabel has been adapted into a patient-facing symptom checker to compete with other products like GP at Hand.

'We're very different to the chatbots, though.' Maude ran me through how apps like Babylon's work. They are constructed from myriad rules; using them is a little like climbing a tree. You start at the trunk – that is the principal symptom, such as fever, or rash, or abdominal pain – and the app presents you with a series of refining questions. Each is like a fork in a branch; the answer you give at every stage influences where you'll eventually end up.

'The problem is,' Maude said, 'you can be asked thirty to fifty questions. Patients get app fatigue and give up. And you have to decide what your most important symptom is – is it the fever, the rash, or the abdominal pain? Only 10% of users have just the one symptom. Pick different principal symptoms and the algorithms take you along completely different trees.'

He demonstrated how the diagnoses the app suggested could vary markedly depending on what a user selected as their most important or worrying symptom. He also explained that every fork in a branch had to have probabilities assigned to it but that these were entirely arbitrary, based purely on the best guesswork of human experts. Small errors at every point could get magnified the further along one went.

Maude's explanations threw light on why the shine was starting to come off symptom checkers like GP at Hand. By that time, my Twitter feed was regularly regaling me with examples where details that any human clinician would instantly recognise as being a potential heart attack, or a breast cancer, failed to register as such on the chatbot. Even Parsa himself, in an interview with the *Daily Telegraph*, admitted that sometimes, 'the AI is just stupid'. And GP at Hand's supposedly stellar performance in the MRCGP exam had subsequently been shown to have been distinctly questionable. The clinical cases it was tested on were presented in highly digested form – ready translated into medical model scenarios, just the sort of material it had been trained to perform on. The app didn't have to do what doctors do all the time: converse with unique human beings, sift and understand their meaning from the words they choose, the silences they leave, the metaphors and similes they employ, and the language their body is also speaking.

As Maude's chatbot tutorial went on, something fundamental became clear. For all the hyped-up talk of AI and deep learning, the symptom checker apps like GP at Hand, with their rules-based branching trees, are merely versions of the same algorithms that underpin NHS Pathways, the software employed so disastrously by NHS 111. The only difference is that Pathways doesn't attempt to make diagnoses. Instead, for a given scenario, it decides on a 'disposition' – what the operator should do to connect the patient with help. As we've seen, in order to mitigate the risk that arises without a firm diagnosis, Pathways routinely overreacts, swamping A&Es and the ambulance service with inappropriate cases. The chatbots can't and don't deal with this problem either. They merely serve up to the user a range of diagnostic possibilities – from the trivial to the urgent – and leave the patient to decide what on earth it is they should do.

Isabel works entirely differently. Maude put it through its paces for me, entering complex case descriptions one minute, and vague symptom clusters the next. The differential diagnoses that appeared virtually instantaneously seemed spot on, and far more comprehensive than I could have come up with unless I'd had a lot more time and potentially done some research. I was impressed.

Curious as to how Isabel would work for someone like Gary, I got Maude to enter his case details. The list Isabel generated contained all the unlikely but serious heart and lung problems that kept eliciting the same 999 ambulance response Gary was habituated to. Nowhere did anxiety feature in the differential. Maude was a bit deflated when I explained. But Isabel shares something in common with all the chatbot apps – it is based purely on the medical model. None is anywhere close to incorporating psychosocial dimensions in their assessments.

Undeterred, Maude wanted to demonstrate Isabel's geographical sensitivities. Fever and gastrointestinal symptoms for a UK resident produced a range of familiar diagnostic possibilities. But when Maude changed the patient's details to indicate recent travel to West Africa, a whole host of tropical diseases were suggested, some of which I had never even heard of. I was impressed all over again. But something niggled.

'Malaria's not there.'

We re-ran the case, altering the symptoms to make them more classic for the parasitic disease. Still the list of diagnoses didn't include malaria. I felt suddenly uncertain; I'd been sure West Africa was malarial but perhaps I'd been wrong. At my suggestion, Maude changed the location to sub-Saharan and, sure enough, up popped malaria high in the differential. I felt extremely embarrassed. I don't do much travel medicine and Isabel was clearly better informed than me. Machine 1, human doc 0.

After our conversation, though, I was left with a nagging doubt. I went to the literature and found I had been right after all: West Africa is of course malarial. What interested me most was how ready I had been to accept that Isabel knew best. Seeing something appear authoritatively on a computer screen has a powerful magic of its own. How would that play out for Gary, I wondered, if next time he gets chest pain and shortness of breath he turns to an AI symptom checker, and is presented with an alarming array of diseases that might be affecting his heart or lungs? Arguably more importantly, what about another patient whose serious pathology isn't recognised by the chatbot of their choice, and who believes the false reassurance?

I emailed Jason Maude to let him know that Isabel had a blind spot about malaria distribution in Africa. He said he would get his team onto it. I discovered there is no capacity for Isabel, or GP at Hand, or any other symptom checker app, to reflect on and learn directly from their mistakes. For that we rely on the humans who design and maintain them.

—

The letter was in the bundle of hospital post I was processing. It was a brief note from A&E concerning a forty-four-year-old patient of ours, David, who had presented with a thunderclap headache. An urgent CT scan had confirmed the suspected diagnosis – a large bleed in the membranes surrounding his brain called a subarachnoid haemorrhage (SAH). He'd been in a bad way. They'd blue-lighted him across to the specialist neurosurgical unit in a neighbouring city where he was currently in a semi-comatose state.

I called his notes up on the computer to code his records. Two things struck me. David had attended the same A&E five days previously with a sudden-onset painful, stiff neck. He'd been told it was muscular and sent away with painkillers. Then he'd consulted with Harriet three days later, complaining of the same thing. I read her notes. She'd come to the identical conclusion as the A&E doctor: that David had muscle spasm. She'd prescribed him stronger pain relief.

Subarachnoid haemorrhage most often arises from the rupture of a swelling in a cerebral artery called an aneurysm. In around half of cases, the SAH is preceded days or even weeks earlier by a sentinel bleed – a small leak of blood that causes an abrupt and unusually severe headache. If a sentinel bleed is correctly diagnosed it presents a window of opportunity in which to perform a procedure to seal the aneurysm and prevent a full-blown SAH from occurring.

With the benefit of hindsight, both Harriet and the A&E doctor had misdiagnosed David's earlier symptoms, which had evidently been a sentinel bleed. The chance to prevent disability or even death had been missed.

Harriet and I reviewed the initial A&E letter and her own notes. It was the absence of headache that had misled her – and presumably our hospital colleague, too. In retrospect, she remembered feeling slightly uneasy at the time, something hadn't quite seemed to fit. But she'd pushed the thought aside and had stuck with the common and seemingly obvious explanation. We sourced some review articles regarding sentinel bleeds and found a range of unusual symptoms that a warning leak might occasionally present with: nausea and vomiting; intolerance of bright light; general feeling of unwellness; or, least common of all, isolated neck pain. No matter that the literature also commented that these nebulous symptoms – so frequently associated with other less serious conditions – were usually misinterpreted by physicians. Harriet was disconsolate.

It couldn't have come at a worse time for her. Some months into her first general practice attachment, her nascent confidence in sifting and sorting undifferentiated presentations had been dealt a huge blow. All doctors, after a missed diagnosis like this, will be affected. For most, it undermines their tolerance of uncertainty. For some time afterwards they will over-investigate and refer much more readily, just in case. This may feel safer but it has negative consequences for patients and the health service alike, putting many patients through unnecessary and potentially harmful investigations and procedures, and adding substantially to hospital workload.

A serious misdiagnosis can be devastating. Harriet kept thinking about David and his family, and couldn't shake the guilt she felt at having – as she saw it – failed them. I told her about the three disasters I've definitely been responsible for since becoming a GP, and gave her the same '10,000 decisions' talk I'd picked up at some point in my career. Ten thousand is the approximate number of meaningful judgements a typical doctor will have to make in a year. Even someone who is 99% perfect will get something wrong 100 times annually. And even if only 1% of those have a serious consequence, we still have to expect a significant incident every year of our working lives. This is inevitable, and the professional response is to reflect honestly, learn any lessons that arise, and take them forward into future practice a bit wiser and a bit more experienced. It didn't help Harriet. Not long afterwards, with David still in a serious condition in hospital, she announced that she wasn't sure she was going to be able to carry on in medicine.

—

Gary did return with Lola and, three weeks into the treatment, he had started to notice marked improvement in his symptoms and his general wellbeing. It was exactly what I'd been hoping for, and opened the door to him beginning to understand his chest pains and breathing difficulties in terms of panic attacks and anxiety. We further explored the difficulties he was contending with and the links between times of heightened stress and aggravated physical symptoms. I prescribed another month's worth of medication and suggested a follow-up appointment. They both nodded, smiling, all trace of hostility and mistrust gone.

I felt buoyed-up by the encounter. After numerous unsatisfactory contacts with health services, I had at last helped Gary make a breakthrough. And it was something no AI would have achieved. Whether Gary had accessed GP at Hand, or Isabel, or 111, the diagnostic possibilities he would have been offered would have focused on the purely physical, and generated yet more anxiety to fan his flames.

That said, were Harriet to have had Isabel installed on her

desktop when David had come to see her, and had she listened to her gut feeling and run his presentation through Isabel's database, the possibility of a sentinel bleed would have been flagged up, along with several other rare, important differentials that only a superhuman familiarity with the medical literature would have suggested. Would it have made a difference? Quite possibly. I have over thirty years' experience yet I hadn't been aware that a sentinel bleed could occasionally present with isolated neck pain. But having that possibility pop up on a computer screen might just have given me pause for thought.

—

I reconnected with Jason Maude in 2021. He'd sent me a new paper from McMaster University in Canada – from where David Sackett had been headhunted back in the 1990s to found the UK's Centre for Evidence-Based Medicine – which showed that use of Isabel increased diagnostic accuracy among both junior and senior clinicians by a small but important percentage. This was Isabel being used for its original purpose, improving the ability of human physicians to get things right in situations where the diagnosis might be obscure.

The worst of Covid had subsided by then so, rather than another remote conversation, I travelled to meet Maude at his Surrey home. One half of his garden office was filled by a wraparound desk with two huge curved-screen PCs from which he steers Isabel's international activities. The other half contained an armchair and a vintage Moto Guzzi 850cc.

The company still markets a patient-facing symptom checker version of Isabel, which has been taken up by patient.info, one of the UK's best health information sites. Maude remains as realistic about its application as he was when we spoke two years previously. As a symptom checker, he sees Isabel's role as an information source for patients – giving them a printout of diagnostic possibilities that could be used to inform their consultations with human physicians. He's never succumbed to the hyperbole to which other health tech entrepreneurs appear prone, that AI will be capable of arriving at definitive diagnoses.

It is a conclusion with which even the likes of IBM would have to agree. IBM set out to create an AI product capable of general diagnosis, which they endearingly named Watson. Despite years of effort and one or two tantalising false dawns, Watson remains as inept as a fresh-faced student on their first day at medical school. As Mark L. Graber, Emeritus Professor of Medicine at Stony Brook University, New York, noted in the editorial accompanying the McMaster paper: 'Diagnosis is likely the most complex cognitive task that humans face.'

It's not just the limitless width of this daunting data landscape – working backwards from ever shifting permutations of just 200 possible symptoms to one of 10,000 possible causes – it's the acquisition of the data itself that defies technological means. The taking of a medical history, the conduct of an examination, are intensely human activities – replete with non-verbal nuances, emotional depths, unique psychosocial circumstances, personality and character, metaphorical and symbolic imagery. The branching chatbot and NHS Pathway trees can never begin to capture even a fraction of the information available to the attentive human eye and ear. Even Isabel, with its impressive ability to turn free text into searchable meaning, can get nowhere near. Then there is the matter of risk. Human doctors rarely arrive at definitive diagnoses, at least not initially. We hold differentials in our minds, subconsciously reordering them constantly as things progress, and forever weighing and balancing the safety or danger attendant on our uncertainties.

Away from the hype over the making of diagnoses, AI is finding its place in medicine. It is, like a stethoscope or a CT scanner, a tool to support doctors, not to replace them. In that respect, IBM were right to christen their project Watson rather than Holmes. When put to work on large sets of narrow data – be they images of skin moles, mammographic X-rays, reams of blood tests, or biopsy specimens – AI engines are superhuman at divining patterns of normality and recognising instances where things subtly deviate. This has the potential to spare radiologists, pathologists and clinicians from having to sift through entire haystacks, instead identifying for them only those things that might prove to be needles.

And AI is demonstrating potential in advancing our understanding and capability. The conundrum of overdiagnosis in cancer screening – those additional tumours that would never go on to cause clinical disease – might prove soluble thanks to computational power. Preliminary results suggest that AI engines have detected patterns of change in tissues adjacent to cancers that predict which require treatment and which can be safely left alone and monitored. As Jason Maude said, computers do very narrow jobs very well.

But to set them to work in one of the broadest jobs of all – making sense of the biopsychosocial world of medicine – will come to be understood as applying a superb technology to precisely the wrong role.

—

David recovered well from his SAH and returned to work and family life, although he has to contend with some residual memory and concentration problems, and a degree of personality alteration. I continued to support Harriet through her crisis of confidence, but it was perhaps her discovery that David attached no blame to her or to the A&E doctor for not recognising his sentinel bleed that was the best medicine. She stayed with her training, passed her MRCGP with distinction, and is now working as a GP in a neighbouring city, gaining in wisdom and experience with every passing year. Like any of us, she feels her responsibility towards patients keenly, and cares deeply if she gets something wrong. The emotional impact from David's case will have made her a better doctor – something that can never be true for a machine.

Gary and Lola didn't keep the next follow-up appointment and haven't been back since. My guess is the stresses have subsided for the moment, but whether it will be me or 111 to whom Gary turns next time he experiences a bad bout of physical symptoms is an open question. Some journeys take a long time to complete, and some never finish at all.

Jason Maude continues to explore applications for Isabel. In the two years since our first encounter, he has developed it into a triaging tool – combining a surprisingly modest set of demographic data with Isabel's differential diagnosis engine to estimate the degree of urgency for a particular patient to seek medical care. It's already been deployed in various US states and other countries but, although it strikes me as being a vast improvement on NHS Pathways and could be a powerful antidote to 111 flooding A&E and the ambulance service with inappropriate cases, the UK is as yet uninterested.

In 2022, Ali Parsa's Babylon began pulling out from providing NHS services. Their business model – based on the notion that their GP at Hand app, backed up if needed by video consultations with doctors, would be able to meet their patients' needs at lower cost – foundered. The hope that technology would reduce the need to employ so many human clinicians proved a fantasy. Yet in March 2022, the right-wing think tank Policy Exchange published *At Your Service*, their vision for the future of general practice. It was accompanied by a commendatory foreword by Sajid Javid, the then Health Secretary, suggesting it was close to government thinking. Policy Exchange envisaged all patient contacts – whether to 111 or GP practices – eventually being routed through something called NHS Gateway where, the hope was, symptom checker apps would divert substantial numbers towards self-help and alternative sources of care. Dressed up in sparkly new terminology, the same tired and discredited tropes are still there.

At the end of my visit, Maude dropped me at the station for my train home. On the way, I asked the question that had lurked in the back of my mind since I first met him, but which I hadn't felt courageous enough to voice before. How did his daughter Isabel – whose critical illness as a toddler inspired Maude to try to remedy the failures that nearly caused her to die – eventually fare? He told me she has needed reconstructive surgery even into adulthood but that she is doing very well, with a thriving career as a management consultant. He gave a wry laugh. 'She's not someone you'd want to cross swords with.' Looking at what her father has created out of inestimable tragedy, that is something I can well understand.

7

MULTIMORBIDITY

Dan was on the phone when I popped my head round the door. He caught sight of me and beckoned me in.

'I was on hold.' He hovered the receiver above the base unit then opened his fingers and let it drop. It spilled off its cradle with a clatter and he had to replace it by hand.

'Trouble?'

He grimaced. 'Sonny Marsden took himself off to see Mike Booth and Mike apparently took one look at him and said, "You've got to go in and get sorted". But of course that'll have to be NHS. And the medics don't want to know.'

I took a seat beside his desk. Sonny was well known to all of us, and it wasn't the first time he'd done something like this. He wasn't wealthy, but he had enough spare cash to seek private appointments with consultants whenever his frustrations with his health problems, and the way the NHS seemed to respond to them, bubbled over.

'Has Mike met him before?'

Dan shook his head. 'Might have done on a post-take round at some point, I'm not sure. But he certainly doesn't know him well.'

I could picture the scene. Mike Booth, one of the many cardiologists at our district general, sitting in the distinctly more rarefied atmosphere of the nearby private hospital undertaking his weekly private practice clinic, only to be confronted by Sonny Marsden. Who would have been short of breath just crossing the room, his bandaged legs grossly swollen, his pulse skittish, his blood pressure awry. I wasn't sure how Sonny got private appointments without a referral, but he always seemed to manage it – maybe he said the letter from his GP was on its way. Whatever it was he told the consultant's private secretary, we never knew anything about it till after the event.

Mike Booth would have made game attempts at taking a history from scratch but I could imagine his mounting despair as Sonny's impenetrably tangled story emerged – the numerous emergency admissions, the palpitations, the breathing difficulty, the ulcerated legs, the chronic back pain, the teetering kidneys, the blood results invariably deranged. And Mike would have tried to establish what medications Sonny was taking and would have been met with tales of multiple adverse drug reactions and completely idiosyncratic dosing regimes. Any suggestion the cardiologist might have made about a change of treatment would have run into a brick wall: 'Tried that before,' Sonny would have said, 'and it damn near killed me. And in any case it was no bloody good.' In the end, the allotted sands having run through the hourglass, Mike would have hoisted a white flag. Sonny needed to be admitted for bed rest and a thorough sort-out, to give Mike the time and monitoring information to try to get to grips with it all.

Only Sonny didn't have insurance. And he'd only had enough money to self-fund a one-off consultation.

'I'll phone your GP, then,' Mike would have said, boxed in by his suggestion of an in-patient stay, 'get you admitted to the Royal.'

Sonny had had any number of spells in an acute NHS bed before. The admitting team would address whatever crisis had arisen – leg sepsis, kidney failure, chest infection – then he would be discharged to out-patient management. Which would result in a flurry of disjointed appointments across various specialties. But after months had passed, punctuated by encounters with harried doctors of varying grades – some of whom would try to find something useful to do, but many of whom would settle for whatever it was that seemed likeliest to get him out of the room – he'd be no further forward. And his frustrations would continue to simmer and stew.

Anyway, at least it didn't look like that was going to happen on this occasion. When Dan had phoned the medical registrar at the overwhelmed Royal, which seemed permanently on a state of black alert, she'd point-blank refused to take Sonny in. It was fair enough. The registrar had grilled Dan as to what the acute problem was supposed to be, and a consultant facing unmanageable complexity in his private clinic was deemed insufficient justification. Sonny's chronic ill-health was not going to be complicated by yet another sojourn on the wards.

'Sonny's up in arms about it,' Dan said.

'So what now?'

'I'm trying to get back in touch with Mike Booth.' He

ran a hand through his hair; he had a million and one other things to do.

'I'll go up there tomorrow,' I said. 'Leave it with me.'

—

Sonny spent most of his life in South London before moving to our area to be near his son following retirement. He'd been a marine engineer. Hanging in the hallway of his warden-assisted flat was the framed commendation he'd won in a design award in the 1980s – I won't pretend to understand the details, but it was something to do with a novel way of constructing hulls. He'd also been an amateur boxer. Next to the engineering prize certificate was a black and white photo of him in singlet and shorts, gloved hands raised and partially obscuring his jaw, posed in the corner of a ring somewhere. He'd have been in his twenties. His eyes were fixed directly on the camera. I wouldn't have wanted to have messed with him back then.

I looked at seventy-year-old Sonny now, sitting across from me semi-recumbent in his recliner chair. His hair, thinned and grey, was swept back in a threadbare semblance of the dark quiff of his youth. His big-boned frame contained echoes of its former power. He was breathing slightly faster than normal just sitting there.

'What about giving furosemide another go?' I said.

'They've never worked for me.'

His legs were lying straight out in front of him, wrapped in bandages below the knees and resting on a couple of large incopads to stop any fluid exudate from staining the upholstery. I contemplated them for a couple of seconds, the shins as thick as the thighs should be, the thighs so swollen they trapped moisture and chafed the skin where they met, such that it was red raw.

'Well, we've got to try something,' I said. 'Bumetanide gives you that awful burning sensation—' he rolled his eyes '—the spironolactone caused nausea—' he nodded '—and you thought bendroflumethiazide made you very ill indeed.' He grimaced at the memory. 'At least we know furosemide doesn't give you any side effects.'

'There's not much point taking something that doesn't do anything, is there?'

'True, true.' I paused for a moment, summoning up the most tactful phrasing I could think of. 'But how were you judging it? Was it by the amount you peed?'

I'd been trying to work with Sonny ever since the last emergency admission – an episode of urinary sepsis from his prostate problems. Looking through his notes I'd had to admit an uncomfortable truth: it wasn't just the hospital that Sonny had a dysfunctional relationship with, it was us, too. His flat was in a sheltered housing complex several miles from surgery. He never came in – taxis would be prohibitive, and his relatives couldn't keep pace with all the hospital stuff, let alone keep bringing him to see his GP. So he relied on home visits, every one of which would take a good hour out of someone's already impossibly time-pressured day. So we'd gradually settled into a reactive pattern, whoever was duty doctor trekking out there whenever a crisis arose, but no single GP taking overall responsibility.

And if the practicalities conspired against frequent follow-up, there was also the small matter of Sonny's health beliefs. The sideboard in his sitting room was rammed with boxes of all the different medications he'd been tried on over the years. It was better stocked than most pharmacies, although I wasn't sure all the drugs were still in date. He was a law unto himself, taking himself off things, putting himself onto others seemingly on a whim. At any given moment it was impossible to know what he was taking, other than it almost certainly wouldn't be what had last been recommended. All the doctors in the surgery had tried engaging with him at one time or another but sooner or later there would be a falling-out – either the doctor would give up, worn down by Sonny's obstreperousness, or Sonny would take against them, ringing reception and demanding that, whoever came next time, it better not be Dr X.

We had to change the game. Despite reception relaying (somewhat gleefully, it must be said) the Anglo-Saxon terms in which Sonny had started to describe me after my first few house calls, I'd kept doggedly visiting. Not that he was anything other than perfectly polite to my face when I got there. And my persistence seemed to be bearing fruit – or if not fruit, at least a bit of blossom. The heart failure Sonny suffered from was very different to the type Simon, my guitar-playing patient in chapter 2, has. Sonny's variety was much more difficult to treat. The only medications that would make any real difference were water tablets (diuretics). And I'd managed to tease out from him the yardstick by which he gauged their effectiveness. If they didn't send him to the loo half a dozen times in the course of a morning then they couldn't be any good. On top of that, if he noticed any symptom, no matter what, in the days after starting a new drug, then the new tablet must be responsible and he would never touch them again.

I reminded him what we'd talked about last time. 'A litre of water weighs a kilogram. Changes in weight are the best way to track how you're getting on.'

I nipped along to his bathroom. He has the full panoply of aids and adaptations – raised loo seat, grab rails, perching stool in the shower, though because of his legs it's been a long time since he's been able to do anything other than a body wash. I retrieved his scales from their home under the sink.

'Let's see where you are today,' I said, rejoining him in the sitting room.

I steadied him as he climbed aboard, placing one elephantine foot then the other on the platform. His distended belly obscured the view, so I crouched down to see where the needle was pointing.

'Seventeen stone,' I said, straightening up and helping him back off again. 'You start with one furosemide every day and I'll come back in two weeks and see how you're getting on.'

—

In October 2011, I was sitting in the Royal Literary and Scientific Institution in Bath, an elegant Georgian building on Queen Square in the heart of the city. I was there for the GP Forum, a monthly meeting of doctors and managers from the twenty-seven practices in our patch. There were around eighty of us assembled in the large upstairs lecture hall, chairs arranged in rows on the varnished wooden floor, the walls crested with ornate cornices, oil portraits of past notables hanging from the picture rails. It was a fine, sunny day outside; the organisers had to lower the blinds partway over the tall sash windows so we could read the slides on the screen at the front of the room.

The RLSI was my favourite setting for the Forum, which, before being scuppered by Covid, rotated around various venues from month to month, the rest of which were bland conference facilities in chain hotels. Wherever it was being held, the meeting followed a familiar agenda. The clinical directors from the district general had the first slot: a briefing on the state of things in the hospital, what different departments were doing to try to get on top of waiting lists, and a chance for them to hear and respond to issues we were encountering with their services. Then various local health and social care managers would take to the floor, outlining and seeking views on new initiatives to improve efficiencies, and tackle pressures and problems in the system. Once the business side of things had been dealt with it was time for the educational component of the afternoon. This usually involved a consultant or other expert being invited to give a presentation about developments in their field, helping us keep up-to-date with advances across the breadth of medical practice.

The speaker that day turned out to be Charlie Berrisford, a GP from one of the city-centre practices. I didn't know him well, but our paths crossed from time to time. I liked him; he was unassuming, somewhere in his mid-forties, with an understated sense of humour. He looked a little awkward as he came to the front, tugging at first one then the other sleeve of his sports jacket. I remember wondering what the topic was going to be.

'When I trained,' he made a show of scanning the room, 'pretty much when *all* of us trained, patients used to die of cancer. Or heart failure. Or stroke. Or some other single, defined disease. And it used to be fairly easy to recognise when they were reaching the end, didn't it? Their liver function would start going off the scale. Or you'd recognise when treatment wasn't holding things any longer. You know the kind of things I mean.'

I did. And it was an arresting start to the talk because it felt like these things still held true. But as Charlie developed his theme I began to see that he was onto something. He painted a picture familiar to every GP in the audience: the usually elderly patient with multiple things wrong with them, lurching from health crisis to health crisis, repeatedly being sent into hospital to be patched up and returned home. Until one time they didn't make it. They'd be stretchered into an ambulance, off-loaded into the strip-lit chaos of A&E, maybe spend hours there on a trolley before, if they were lucky, making it to a ward. Only then to die.

This was what was exercising Charlie, the fact that we were very poor at predicting when these kinds of patients were approaching the end of life. When looking after someone with a disease like metastatic cancer, we were all too familiar with its typical course. It allowed us to instigate important conversations – to ensure they'd got their affairs in order, encourage them to do things and see people important to them in their remaining time, and to think about where they would want to be when they died – usually, but not invariably, at home. Difficult but vital discussions could be had, addressing resuscitation status and the desirability or otherwise for hospital admission in the event of deterioration. The ambulance service and GP out-of-hours could be informed so they knew what to do in a crisis at night or over a weekend. District nurses and hospice input could be arranged, support for family provided, just-in-case injectable drugs lodged in their home to allow a quick response to rapid changes in symptoms. We could put in place everything to make death as dignified, and as in accordance with the patient's wishes, as possible.

What Charlie was alerting us to – and he was the first person I heard articulate it so explicitly – was that fewer and fewer of our patients any longer fitted this paradigm. Our treatments across the whole gamut of medicine minimise damage, slow progression, alleviate symptoms, allow life to go on for years and years. Patients are routinely surviving conditions that would once have been life-limiting. Unarguably a good thing. Yet the longer life goes on, the more other things go wrong. Pathology piles on pathology, further complicated by the declines associated with advanced ageing. Such patients had certainly been around when I was training but they were encountered only infrequently. Charlie presented data to show that over the preceding twenty years, the prevalence of chronic diseases – things that can't be cured but are instead lived alongside – had more than doubled. And the numbers of patients with four or more such concurrent conditions had trebled.

Patients like this tend not to die of any one thing. Death, when it comes, is more akin to a house of cards collapsing. Arthritic joints lead to immobility and the use of painkillers, which might cause an already weakened bowel to become constipated, in turn precipitating a urinary tract infection. This can send the patient 'off legs' and create delirium, fluid intake drops off as they no longer recognise the need to drink, and dehydration causes their kidneys to fail.

The scenario outlined above can be rectified relatively easily and in many circumstances it would be appropriate to do so. It's the bread and butter of acute admission: intravenous fluids to reverse dehydration, antibiotics to treat sepsis, frequent bloods to monitor and guide correction of kidney failure. But for a patient in the last weeks of life from an advanced cancer, for example, someone who wants to be at home surrounded by family – all you're going to achieve in that situation is to condemn them to spend their final hours or days on a noisy, chaotic hospital ward, if not on a trolley in a corridor in A&E.

And that was Charlie's point. It is easy enough to know when to shift our focus onto palliative care in a patient in whom our training allows us to identify that they are approaching the end of life. But how do we achieve the same holistic outcomes for the kinds of patients we increasingly see? How do we recognise the point at which medical heroics cease to be helpful and actually cause harm in someone who doesn't have a single terminal disease?

—

Sonny's daughter-in-law, Maria, let me in. She had a tea towel in one hand.

'How are things?'

She turned her mouth down. 'Oh, you know.'

Sonny was propped semi-upright on an array of cushions and pillows. The room was cramped, his double bed occupied the majority of the floor space, leaving corridors of carpet round three sides that were barely wide enough to accommodate his walking frame. The side table was cluttered with beakers and a water jug and some kind of drinks maker for brewing cups of tea.

'How are you doing?' I said.

He gave me a lopsided grin. 'Better than I was.'

I perched on the edge of the bed and put my medical bag down. 'So what happened?'

'Bloody kidneys.'

I already knew what had happened medically – the discharge summary had told me. Eddie and Maria had called round at the weekend and found him drowsy and confused. The ambulance had taken him in. His admission bloods had shown his renal function to have plummeted to a quarter of where it had been – and it hadn't been all that great to start with.

'Sure. But how did it happen, is what I mean.'

Sonny shrugged his shoulders.

'He wasn't drinking anything.' Maria's voice came from the doorway behind me.

Sonny shot her a look and she turned and disappeared, but the damage had been done. Over the course of ten minutes or so, I prised the story out of him. It turned out it wasn't a recent thing. Unbeknownst to any of us, Sonny had long been trying to manage his heart failure with fluid restriction. It seemed to make sense, if his legs were waterlogged then you'd think you'd want to stop tipping so much of it in the top end.

'Used to do it all the time before weigh-ins,' he told me, sounding rueful. I thought back to him standing on the scales. And that black and white picture in the hall: singlet and shorts, gloved hands raised in front of his face.

'It's not a boxing match,' I said.

Actually, Sonny could be forgiven for having latched on to fluid restriction as a way of trying to help. Until relatively recently, heart-failure patients would often be advised to limit intake to less than two litres a day. But the evidence for it turned out not to stack up. Indeed, what trials exist suggest it makes people feel worse while rarely conferring any benefit. The internet is still littered with outdated advice, though.

'I wasn't doing anything different.'

'You were with the furosemide, though, weren't you?'

He nodded glumly. With Sonny running himself on the dry side, adding a regular diuretic – as opposed to an erratic tablet here or there which had been his traditional modus operandi – must have upset a precarious balance. Flow of blood into the kidneys is regulated by complex mechanisms and rather than encouraging water output as intended, Sonny suddenly taking regular diuretics while simultaneously dehydrating himself had tipped things the other way.

'What do I do about all these?'

He reached across to the other bedside table and passed me an untidy pile of identical opened envelopes. I recognised the hospital franking mark. While an in-patient he'd had an ultrasound of his kidneys, which had picked up an incidental finding of a dangerous swelling of the main artery running through the abdomen – an aortic aneurysm. His blood tests had shown up the anaemia I'd already been keeping an eye on. His leg ulcers – stubbornly non-healing despite our district nurses' best efforts – had been a cause for concern. Then there were the palpitations, and the attacks of breathing difficulty that his inhalers didn't help. He'd had no fewer than six out-patient follow-ups arranged – cardiology, respiratory, dermatology, vascular surgery, gastroenterology plus a CT scan. How many would his son – or more likely Maria – be willing or able to take him to? For how many would he have to cast himself on the mercies of patient transport? But one way or another presumably he thought he'd better get to them. Six appointments. The hospital must think there's a hell of a lot wrong. And there is a hell of a lot wrong.

'Let's talk them through.'

I've seen many examples like this, but Sonny's was one of the most egregious. It will all have been with the best of intentions. The junior doctors on the ward will have been hard-pressed and overburdened, and keen to get Sonny back out to make his bed available again. So they'd have uncritically followed protocol. Aortic aneurysm: refer vascular surgery. Non-healing leg ulcers: add dermatology. Unexplained anaemia: one for gastroenterology. Weird palpitations: ask cardiology. Asthma in the mix: better involve respiratory. There must presumably have been a consultant involved, but even that hadn't stopped the scattergun from firing. Increasing specialisation means there are few generalists left in secondary care, most people stick rigidly within their narrow field of expertise and spin-pass other problems elsewhere. And the pressure to discharge patients quickly favours snap decisions, postponing time-consuming discussions, a bit like kicking a can down the road.

I outlined for Sonny what was likely to happen in each scenario. How his poor health would make major surgery or invasive investigations too risky, so for many of the appointments he would attend – with all the upheaval and difficulty each day at the hospital would involve – he would simply be told to leave things alone. 'The aneurysm,' I said, 'may never pose you any problem. If it did at any point, well. But trying to fix it, that would be pretty much guaranteed to cause you harm.'

It took quite some time to talk it all through. He called Maria in for a second pair of ears, too. In the end he decided to cancel several of the clinic appointments. There were a couple he thought might be of use.

'I don't know,' he said, gesticulating at his tree-trunk legs, the incopads. 'It's like I can feel them filling up.' He shook his head slowly. 'And then my breathing gets worse, and my heart goes nineteen to the dozen. My inhaler doesn't help. Even the water tablets don't do anything either. It must be my heart.' He let his hand fall limply by his side. 'It feels like I'm dying.'

—

The GP Forum at which Charlie Berrisford spoke was just over ten years ago. That feels barely credible. At the time, there were no commonly understood terms to encapsulate what Charlie was describing. Yet today the two words that describe these phenomena are so embedded in the medical lingua franca that they feel like they've been with us for ever. Multimorbidity. Frailty.

Multimorbidity seems easy enough to understand: the coexistence of many different diseases. Yet it is much more than that. Diseases interact, overlap, complicate and aggravate each other. Sonny's chronic oedema from heart failure has caused permanent damage to his legs such that they will never now drain or return to normal. The altered tissues are prone to ulceration, and impaired healing means this may very well remain. The breached skin leaves him susceptible to infection, and episodes of sepsis put his ailing heart under still further strain. Drugs that might help his heart aggravate his asthma, others to ward off stroke compound anaemia that in turn aggravates numerous bodily functions. Trying to control his blood pressure to protect heart, aortic aneurysm and kidney function leaves him prone to falls. And his precarious kidneys can at any time turn helpful drugs into killers. And so it goes on.

Frailty is a related concept, organs and systems in the body losing more and more reserve capacity with both disease and advancing age. Muscles thin and become weaker, impairing balance, strength and mobility. Elsewhere, organs like the bladder and bowel begin to malfunction and fail. Lung function diminishes, decompensating breathlessness from other causes. The vigour of the immune response pales, infection can quickly become overwhelming. The ageing brain loses memory, coordination and cognitive acuity, and sensations like hunger and thirst, which usually ensure nutrition and hydration, become blunted.

The challenges of multimorbidity and frailty go beyond the problem Charlie Berrisford identified a decade ago: how to recognise the impending end of life in complex, multifactorial states. Charlie proposed a rule of thumb: would you be surprised if this person were to die in the next six months, or maybe the next year? There are no reductive ways to analyse and break that down, but if the answer, based on extensive experience and formed of gut instinct is No, then it is time to be starting discussions about palliation and advance care planning, just as we would when recurrent cancer has begun to take hold.

But these are circumstances that the NHS still struggles to adapt to. Our whole system was constructed in the era of single diseases. Hospital care remains overwhelmingly geared towards managing discrete episodes. Increasing specialisation and grinding time pressure mean it's rare for anyone to take a properly holistic view. GPs, alongside geriatricians and paediatricians, are the only generalists left. And our list sizes are entirely outdated – the average GP is currently trying to look after 2,200 patients. There's scant room for the complexity of multimorbidity, frailty and the ensuing polypharmacy to be properly overviewed.

—

Dan put the letter in my pigeonhole – he'd scrawled 'One for you, I think!' across the top.

There'd been a certain amount of good-natured teasing among the team over my status as Sonny's lead GP. Most had tried it at some point, only to be ground down in one way or another, and the expectation was that sooner or later I would go the same way. But gradually Sonny and I had been building an understanding. The banter fizzled out as the team noticed how things had improved. Sonny's frequent requests for urgent visits had all but dried up. If he did ring for attention between scheduled visits, it was me he asked for. There was still the occasional quip from colleagues, mock sympathy for the bed I'd made for myself – the repeated house calls took a significant time toll. I kept saying that I didn't expect things between Sonny and me to remain rosy indefinitely. But secretly I was pleased. I seemed to have made some headway.

Now this. The letterhead of Jake Lazarides, yet another of the local cardiologists. Sonny was well known to Jake, under whose care he'd often come within the NHS. So Jake hadn't been thrown the way Mike Booth was when Sonny turned up in his private practice clinic. Indeed, he'd seen Sonny a few times before on a paid-for basis. He'd taken things in his stride to the extent of not suggesting a further admission.

Even so. He planned to throw the cardiological book at him. Another echocardiogram. Holter monitoring of heart rhythm over a prolonged period. Radionucleotide stress test for occult angina. And recommendations for an additional drug, a variation on a theme that Sonny had previously tried and discarded as no good.

I didn't blame Jake. They were all, in one respect, perfectly logical things to do. Faced with a patient sat in front of you, there feels an imperative to do something. And if you're a cardiologist, years steeped in that discipline will lead you to interpret symptoms from a cardiological point of view. Sonny's heart failure was of a type only really responsive to diuretics. But reinvestigating might turn up something new. The palpitations and breathless attacks could represent bouts of rhythm disturbance. And maybe Sonny did have areas of heart muscle that weren't being adequately supplied with oxygen. But I was far from convinced. At least, given Sonny's constrained resources, Jake was going to get all these done under the NHS. Nothing was going to happen quickly. And although it felt like a setback – Sonny taking himself back for yet another opinion – I thought there was a way I might turn the situation into something good.

'You're in his bad books again,' Liz on reception said, her eyes laughing. I was scanning the visit book at the end of morning surgery. Sonny Marsden's name was in there. 'He said – in no uncertain terms – it wasn't to be you.'

I didn't ask for elaboration, but I could imagine the kind of language Sonny would have employed. 'I know what it's about,' I told her. It would be easier to leave it for a colleague – that was, after all, what Sonny said he wanted, and I felt uncomfortable appearing to ride roughshod over his wishes. But it would just perpetuate the patterns we'd all become locked into. 'It's me that's got to go.'

I pulled up outside his flat a little later, having first moved the parking cone that the warden placed in the empty space to discourage unauthorised use. Maria was there again to let me in. She was dressed smartly in navy skirt and jacket and noticeably made up, as though going on somewhere for lunch or a meeting.

'He's in the lounge,' she told me. Neither her expression nor tone gave me much clue.

'It's the B team again,' I said to Sonny. He was in the recliner chair, remote control in hand, his swollen legs protruding from under a tartan blanket.

'Oh, hello.' He muted the telly. 'I hoped it might be you.'

I never blow the receptionists' cover – far better that he can express his feelings unguardedly, so I know what's going on with his mood. I pulled a pouffe over and squatted down beside his chair.

'So I got the letter from Dr Lazarides,' I said. 'If you wanted to discuss it with someone else we can arrange that. But I thought it might be something we should talk through.'

'Are you pissed off with me?'

I laughed. 'Sonny, it's completely up to you what you do. Was it helpful?'

He lifted the remote control and peered at it as if suddenly struck by something about the buttons. 'He wants to do more tests. And what's that other tablet he's on about? Is it a beta blocker again?'

'Yes, but another one that only acts on the heart. He thinks it might help the palpitations.'

'It'll upset my asthma.'

'We don't know that. It shouldn't. Do you want to give it a go?'

He laid the remote down on the blanket. 'OK. In the lowest dose.'

'Sure, we can do that.'

I checked his pulse rate and was getting my blood pressure cuff out of my bag.

'What about those tests?' He shifted position in the chair, wincing from his back pain.

'He obviously thinks they'll help.'

He stayed silent while I took his blood pressure. I listened to the Korotkoff sounds, the rhythmic thuds as blood begins to pulse again through the compressed artery, which I must have done countless thousands of times over my career. The cuff steadily deflated, air escaping the valve with a soft hiss. It's so hard to know how to turn the conversation onto what really counts. It's much easier to follow a patient's cue. But Sonny wasn't going to do that, not on his own. I took my stethoscope out of my ears, removed the blood pressure cuff with a Velcro rip.

'I'll be off now,' Maria called from the doorway. 'See you Saturday.'

'Thanks, love.' He waved a hand but she'd already gone. The front door clunked shut behind her.

'It's doing it again!' He looked like he was wincing but he hadn't moved. His breathing had quickened visibly. I laid a hand on his wrist: his pulse was a bit faster but not dramatically so.

'Have you got pain?'

He shook his head. 'I can't breathe.'

He could though. I listened into his chest: crackles in the bases but nothing new. His respirations slowed a bit even as I examined him.

'Should I use the inhaler?'

'Is that what you'd usually do?'

He nodded. His face still looked drawn.

'It's settling, Sonny. I think it's going to calm down.'

And it did, whatever it was, over the next minute or two.

'Fuck's sake.' He put his hand to his chest, shaking his head. 'It's got to be my heart, hasn't it?'

'Do you know what?' I eased my stethoscope off and laid it round my neck. 'I really don't think so.'

—

Charlie Berrisford's talk has stayed with me in the way paradigm-shifting things do – his rough and ready remedy for breaking the dispiriting loop of multimorbidity and frailty, patients trapped in ever more intervention and medicalisation when we ought instead to be helping them plan for a dignified natural end to their life. Ask yourself a simple question, Charlie had said: would I be surprised if this patient were to die within the next six months, within the next year? There may be no single disease present whose terminal course is familiar to us, but we know from all we've experienced when the cumulative toll on a single body begins to overwhelm. If the answer is yes, I would be surprised, then it's right to keep staging attempts at rescue. But if the answer is no, then it's time to do something else.

Maria may have closed the front door behind her but she'd opened another one in Sonny's living room. I suddenly twigged what it was I'd seen on Sonny's face.

'Do you feel frightened?' I asked him.

He looked at me for a long moment. He made to speak a couple of times but stopped. 'Not of dying,' he said eventually. 'I'm ready to go.' He waved a hand vaguely. 'Not much of a life anymore, is it, stuck here like this.'

'I think that was panic – the palpitations and breathing.'

He gave a sharp exhalation through his nose. 'You might be onto something. What though?'

'I don't know. What was going through your mind?'

There was another long pause, Sonny periodically shaking his head as though having a silent argument with himself.

'What if she comes in and finds me? You know. Days after.'

—

I referred Sonny to our care coordinator, who sorted out daily visits from a carer, ostensibly to help him with washing and dressing. The greatest value to Sonny was that, when he came to die, it would likely be a paid professional who discovered him, not his daughter-in-law, and not after his body had begun to decompose. He decided against pursuing Jake Lazarides's gamut of investigations. I kept thinking back to that black and white photo in his hall, Sonny as pugilist. All his life he'd been a fighter. Now, at last, he was ready to let go.

Part Three

TWENTY-FIRST-CENTURY DOCTORS

8

THE ICE MAN COMETH

Jim was tall and lean, with a mellifluous Northern Irish accent and a confident manner. He'd been attached to the surgery just a matter of weeks and already he'd charmed the entirety of the reception, admin and nursing teams – and several of the female doctors to boot.

I do a joint surgery with my registrars on Thursday mornings. We take turn about, me giving feedback on their consultations and them watching me in action for the others. Both are equally valuable. I get to highlight when things have gone well for them and advise on ways to improve. Observing me, they pick up tips and techniques that would otherwise take them years to refine. And when one of my consultations turns out less than ideally I can model reflection and self-directed learning – as well as reassuring by example that perfection is never an attainable goal.

Jim listened to me making the first phone call to Darren, who wanted to talk about his nine-month-old son, Harry, and his reaction to certain foods. 'He gets these swollen lips and rash on his face any time he has tomato – huge they are, his lips, and the skin round his mouth goes all red and sore – then he had something with egg in it for tea the other day and – oh I don't know – he didn't get the lip thing or the rash or anything but he was sick and in terrible pain drawing his knees up like he had bellyache all night.'

Darren's speech was pressured, the words tumbling out almost on top of each other. I was scrolling through Harry's notes as he talked. None of this was new. The health visitors had already put in a referral to the paediatric allergy team and the dieticians. And they'd advised Darren and Lisa to avoid giving either tomato or egg until the situation had been clarified. I could hear Harry burbling in the background. Darren might even have had him in his arms, he sounded that close. He certainly sounded very happy.

'It must be scary,' I said, 'having Harry react like this.'

'It is, doc, it really is. We just don't know what to give him. It's like we're just sitting here waiting for the next bomb to explode.'

The health visitor had last seen Harry ten days ago, following the reaction to egg. She'd advised them to stick to the foods Harry had proven himself to be all right with while the situation got sorted out. I checked with Darren that this is what they'd been doing. 'So has anything happened since then?' I asked.

'No, no, he's been fine. It's just it's doing our heads in.'

I couldn't work out what I was supposed to do. 'I can hear it's very stressful. How's Lisa coping?'

'She's out with friends at the moment.'

Suddenly I had an inkling.

'She's struggling, is she?'

There was a long exhalation at the other end of the line. 'I can see the sense in it, honestly. Just stick with what we know is OK till he's been up the hospital. But she's gone to pieces. She can't even bring herself to feed him anymore, even if it's something he's had loads of times. It's not just meals. She's pretty much stopped having anything to do with him.'

I had a sudden vision of where she might be right then as I was talking to Darren – I'm not sure why, but I pictured her walking in a park, her head bowed, a friend either side of her, supportive arms on her back, her shoulders, leaning in attentively as she cried and tried to speak.

'What does she say about it?'

'That's just it,' he said. 'If I try and talk to her, it just blows up in a row.'

'That sounds really difficult. Listen. This is what I think we should do.'

Debriefing afterwards, Jim said he realised he had a lot to learn. He'd been entirely focused on the allergy problem and had been wracking his brain throughout the first part of the call: what would he advise had he been conducting the consultation? What other foodstuffs ought they to avoid lest they trigger a cross-reaction in Harry? Might there be a role for antihistamines pending paediatric review? Now he could see what the real issues were – a couple in meltdown, and both in need of the urgent support and follow-up I'd promised to arrange. The more we'd got to the heart of the matter, the more Darren's speech had calmed.

Jim and I swapped seats. The next consultation was face-to-face. Deepti, a facilities manager with the local water company in her late forties, whom Jim had triaged the previous day. Jim was more experienced than many registrars, he'd spent three years doing A&E in Australia between his foundation programme and returning to the UK to do post-graduate training in general practice. He smiled and gestured for her to take a seat once he'd brought her through from the waiting room.

'So you've got this cough, you said?' he started. 'Remind me, how long's it been going on?'

Deepti looked well enough in herself. 'Two weeks – but actually it's starting to get a bit better. I'm still getting sweats in the night, though.'

'Is there anything coming off the chest?'

'No, no, it's a dry cough – it always has been. I'm sure it's just a virus. But I'm exhausted.' She put a hand up to her neck.

'And your breathing's OK? Any chest pain? Runny nose? Sore throat?'

'No, nothing like that. I'm just so tired.'

Jim rattled through a whole load of other negatives then checked if it was all right to examine her. Temperature, pulse, respirations, oxygen saturations all normal. He listened to her breathing, his stethoscope methodically alighting on upper, middle and lower zones.

He sat back in his chair. 'And what did you think was wrong?'

Deepti looked a bit taken aback. 'That's why I came to the doctor!'

Jim chuckled, and I knew he meant it reassuringly. 'I think you're right – it is just a virus. And I think you're well on the mend.'

He made a few closing remarks and told her to come again if it wasn't all fully better in a couple more weeks. He asked if she had any questions, to which Deepti gave a shake of her head and said, 'No, it's fine'. She put her jacket back on and we all exchanged goodbyes.

I let Jim type up his notes after she'd left.

'So why did she come?' I asked, when he'd finished.

He looked at me quizzically. 'Because she's got a cough?'

'It was getting better. She said that.'

'I don't know,' he said. 'Was she worried it was Covid? Or maybe she thought she needed antibiotics?'

I smiled. 'We don't know, do we? That's the point. What *was* she worried about? What did she think we could do to help?'

Jim looked a bit chastened. I hastened to reassure him.

'It's not that you've done anything wrong, as such. But think about that last case, the baby with the food allergies.'

I let him have a few seconds to ponder.

'Take them together,' I told him, 'that one and this. They're a brilliant example of the importance of patient-centred consulting.'

—

Peter Tate came outside to greet me before I'd made it as far as his front gate.

'Phil, welcome!' he called. 'Very good to see you.'

His voice was as I remembered, the remnants of a Newcastle accent lending it a rich colour. And his round face, pudgy frame and amused blue eyes still made him seem the embodiment of bonhomie. We'd kept in touch by email and Christmas cards but it had been sixteen years since I'd last seen him. That had been at a meal attended by a dozen of his former registrars to mark his retirement at the age of fifty-six on health grounds.

'We're in the garage, I'm afraid,' he explained, as he led me through the garden at the side of the house. 'The plan was to eat out here. But British summers!' He laughed. The foliage and flowers were bowed and bedraggled by the rain that had been falling all morning.

He let me in a side door into the brick-built garage. The walls were lined with motley free-standing shelving units laden with plastic storage containers, tins of paint, vases, stools, an incongruously large pestle and mortar. One of the many cardboard boxes had 'Country Rose tea set' scrawled on it in marker pen. It had been three years since Peter and Judith had moved to Poundbury from their five-bedroom cottage in Corfe Castle. The downsizing was ongoing.

'Judy sends her apologies,' Peter said, ushering me towards the area of floor space he'd cleared that morning to make room for a round table draped with a striped cotton tablecloth. 'Even yesterday she was still up for it, but there was something on TV last night and she lost her nerve.'

This was summer 2020, the lull between the first and second Covid waves. Vaccines were still nothing more than a distant hope. Judith has brittle type 1 diabetes. Even though case numbers were rumbling at a low level, there'd been a documentary highlighting that the virus was still very much in circulation, particularly in healthcare settings. If anyone were to bring it into the carefully shielded Tate home it was going to be someone like a practising GP.

Peter laid out the plates of bruschetta and bowls of salads, and checked I wanted nothing beyond sparkling water to accompany mine. The first time I'd met him, back in 1992, things had been somewhat different. I'd turned up for my interview in suit and tie. He'd met me in the practice lobby, straight from doing phone calls after morning surgery, shaken my hand heartily and announced he was taking me for a pint and a pie.

I knew I wanted to be his registrar almost immediately, a conviction that only grew stronger the longer we chatted over my CV in the pub. I'd mentioned I was a runner and it turned out Peter had been one, too. 'I used to find it great thinking time, just rolling along mile after mile.' He smiled a bit wistfully. 'I don't get to do it these days, mind.' He also wanted to talk about my writing. I'd started doing short stories as a medical student, and had taken a year off before starting GP training to have a stab at a novel. Peter was enthusiastic, seeing it as a healthy counterbalance. Many of the other prospective trainers I'd been to visit thought my literary interests were decidedly suspect, indicating a lack of seriousness about medicine. Peter told me he was also an author. Around ten years previously, he'd co-written, with three other researchers, a book called *The Consultation: An Approach to Learning and Teaching*. What he didn't say at the time was that he was far from content with the limited academic readership a book like that was only ever going to reach.

The interview, refreshingly informal, went well. This was where I wanted to come, I firmly decided, and Peter said he'd be happy to have me. There would be two more years of hospital posts to complete first, but after that I would spend the final twelve months of my training programme as his registrar at Marcham Road. And while I was busy gaining further experience in paediatrics, obstetrics and gynaecology, dermatology, palliative care, neurological rehabilitation and psychiatry up at John Radcliffe Hospital, Peter was to write a slim publication that was to have an outsized impact on the medical world.

—

Medically speaking there was nothing wrong with Jim's consultation with Deepti. In fact, it conformed to the kind of encounters that have gone on between doctors and patients from time immemorial. Jim was in the role his training had groomed him for, the professional with expertise. Deepti, to him, was the supplicant, come to seek his opinion about the nature of her disease.

The history he'd obtained had pointed strongly towards a self-limiting infection. Nothing about his subsequent examination had suggested otherwise. Ninety-nine times out of a hundred – more, even – the passage of time would prove him right. Deepti's cough would fully resolve, her night sweats would fizzle out, her energy would finally return. And even if this did turn out to be one of those rare occasions when there was something unsuspected going on, Deepti would fail to get better and would soon consult again. That would be the time to arrange blood tests and a chest X-ray. It would be neither possible nor appropriate to do that for every patient presenting as Deepti had, on the off-chance the initial diagnosis might ultimately prove to be wrong.

What's hard to appreciate sitting in a GP surgery is that, for every patient like Deepti, there will be numerous others with the same symptoms who don't seek medical advice. Something had happened to make her think twice. Maybe a work colleague had come down with a similar illness and when he'd been to his doctor he'd been told he needed treatment with antibiotics. Or it could be that, given that her cough was resolving, the persistence of fatigue and night sweats was starting to cause Deepti concern. Perhaps, when she'd discussed things with friends, it had sparked comments that she might be entering the menopause. Maybe they'd reminded her of the university contemporary she remembered who'd been diagnosed with HIV. Trying to sort out these conflicting theories she may have turned to Dr Google, only to find mention of other threatening possibilities like lymphoma. Eventually, her mind teeming with imponderables, anxiety starting to disrupt her sleep, she would have turned to the person able to help, her GP.

And it could be that Jim's confident and unconcerned opinion would have been all it took to put her at ease. Oftentimes that would be true. But Deepti would also know from newspaper headlines and viral posts on social media that doctors are far from infallible. Quite possibly Jim's breezy 'come back in a couple of weeks if it's not all better' could have been exactly what she'd heard other doctors had said to patients in whom they were subsequently found to have initially not made an important diagnosis. How was she even to know that the scenarios causing her to lose sleep had actually crossed Jim's mind, that he'd considered and discounted them? What if one or more of them simply hadn't occurred to him?

At the very least, she would be in for an anxious couple of weeks waiting to see if, as predicted, everything would resolve. In the meantime, she might return again and again to the internet, scouring web pages and forums, seeking ever more information in an attempt to assure herself that the doctor had been right. And every night that she woke up with sweat-dampened pyjamas, every afternoon as she struggled to keep going despite startling fatigue, would have served to undermine her confidence.

Or Deepti's decision to consult Jim might have had nothing to do with diagnosis. What if she were also sure it was a self-limiting illness, but it was simply taking too much of a toll? Maybe she'd hoped Jim would pick up on her continuing fatigue and suggest signing her off for a couple of weeks to allow her time to recuperate. Or perhaps there'd been an incident – she'd missed something in the course of her work that she ought to have picked up on, an oversight she attributed to having been unwell. Getting a consultation documented in her medical records might have felt to her like an insurance policy in case of a future disciplinary action.

We could speculate endlessly. The point was, Jim hadn't established why she'd come, so he had no idea whether or not he'd met her needs. And neither had Deepti – an articulate, educated professional – volunteered the information herself, not even after Jim asked her what she thought was wrong, nor when he gave her a chance to ask any questions at the end. Some patients will speak out, but they are in the minority. Many people fear appearing impertinent, they don't want to come across as telling the doctor how to do their job. Others are acutely embarrassed, reluctant to reveal their anxieties in case they're thought to be ludicrous. Still others will be subconsciously superstitious, fearing that if they say the word 'cancer' out loud then it would be bound to make it come true.

—

Peter Tate began his GP career in the late 1970s, taking up a partnership in a market town just outside Oxford. Shortly afterwards, he began to suffer episodes of collapse. He was admitted to hospital for investigation and, as a by-product, gained a first-hand appreciation of quite how badly doctors of the era communicated. The ward round would appear, murmured conversations would take place at the foot of the bed, opinions and information would be dispensed, then the ward round would move on. No one was interested in eliciting, let alone addressing, the fears and uncertainties Peter had about the heart condition with which he'd been diagnosed.

Just as striking to him was the impact he observed among his fellow in-patients. After the consultant and his retinue had departed, Peter would listen to their conversations. They all had dreads and beliefs concerning their respective illnesses, about which the doctors charged with caring for them were oblivious. Peter could see the yawning gulf between what his white-coated colleagues were doing – which they would have felt was an eminently good medical job – and what he and his fellow patients needed. He left hospital with a cardiac pacemaker in situ and a determination to do something to change the culture of medicine.

His opportunity came shortly afterwards with the arrival at Oxford University of psychologist David Pendleton. Pendleton was keen to conduct research in the developing field of doctor–patient communication, and recruited Peter and two other GP trainers, Theo Schofield and Peter Havelock, to analyse many hundreds of recorded consultations conducted by a cohort of experienced GPs. What they found was striking. While most of the doctors were fulfilling the time-honoured, paternalistic role of the physician – arriving at a medical diagnosis and prescribing treatment and/or giving a prognosis to an essentially passive patient – around 10% had honed a completely different style. They were interested in the sense that their patients made of their symptoms and situations, and they employed various techniques to draw this information out. Having understood their patients' perspectives, they were able to answer important questions such as 'What has led this person to consult about this problem at this point in time?', as well as to get a sense of how much or little overlap there might be between the patients' health beliefs and the way a physician would view things. Not only did this equip them to make more nuanced and holistic diagnoses, they were also able to tailor their explanations, advice and management to the individual in front of them. An individual who, crucially, had been fully involved in the whole process.

The four researchers wrote up their findings in *The Consultation.* One of the key concepts they articulated was ICE – that was Peter's brainchild, a snappy mnemonic for the powerful 'ideas, concerns and expectations' about their illness that a patient has invariably formed prior to consulting a professional. It was these ideas, concerns and expectations that remained hidden in the majority of medical consultations, yet which created vastly more meaningful encounters – for both patient and doctor – when they were successfully unearthed. But in the ten years following publication of *The Consultation* what felt to Peter like vital concepts to change the way medicine was practised had remained frustratingly confined to the academic ivory tower.

It was a beer at The George in Sutton Courtenay in 1993

that was to change that. A friend of Peter's, Andrew Bax, was leaving a long stint at Blackwell's to set up his own publishing firm, Radcliffe Press, with a focus on medical titles. Andrew was attracted by the fresh thinking Peter's ICE idea represented. By the time the pair had drained their first pint Andrew had commissioned Peter to write about it for him – a book directed principally at the new generation of doctors who, like me, had yet to fix their consulting style and who would be more receptive to novel thinking. The only thing was, Andrew was in a hurry to get his title list together. He wanted Peter's book pretty damn quickly.

Peter rose to the challenge, writing *The Doctor's Communication Handbook* in under a fortnight – the bulk of it over the course of just one weekend – crouched at his Amstrad computer loaded with the prototypical word processor, LocoScript. All the material was crammed in his head. He'd been pondering and refining it for years. He imagined his then registrar, a doctor named Mark Mayall, sitting beside him – he wrote as if expounding his ideas over the course of an extended tutorial. It worked. Reading it was like having Peter talking to you there in the room. On publication in 1994, *The Doctor's Communication Handbook* garnered excellent reviews and was highly commended in the *British Medical Journal*'s Book of the Year award. By the time I joined Peter's practice as his next trainee that autumn, his book was on every GP registrar's recommended reading list.

Not content with reaching a far wider audience, Peter pushed hard – in collaboration with several other progressive GPs – for the Royal College of General Practitioners

(RCGP) to formally incorporate what had become known as 'consultation skills' into the training curriculum. Now, as well as learning about the diagnosis and management of the myriad diseases a GP will encounter, young doctors throughout the country would be taught the necessity of discovering and engaging with each individual patient's unique perspectives. And on the basis that if people are going to be tested on something they will pay it due attention, Peter – an examiner with the RCGP – led the complex process of devising methods of assessing those skills as part of the college's membership qualification. For many years this involved registrars submitting video recordings of a series of sample consultations from their day-to-day practice. This approach gave way to the Clinical Skills Assessment and its latter-day variant the Simulated Consultation Assessment, both of which test the same competencies under examination conditions using actors to roleplay carefully devised clinical encounters.

—

Just like Jim, in those opening minutes of the call with Darren I'd focused exclusively on Harry's food allergies. That had so obviously been what Darren wanted to talk about. Only the longer it went on, the less sure I'd become.

How did we get to what the problem actually was? It started with that niggling sense that I didn't know what I was expected to do. I might have assumed I knew Darren's ideas and concerns – something about his baby having multiple food reactions, and worrying what might happen if/when Harry encountered the next unsuspected allergen

– but the health visitors had all that in hand, so my assumptions would have been wrong. And I certainly didn't have a clue about Darren's expectations. Put it another way, I couldn't even begin to answer the question: why has this dad phoned about this problem at this point in time?

Uncovering ICE, the patient's ideas, concerns and expectations, is easy when the patient is aware of what they are and is happy to vocalise them. Most of the time they are far more opaque. I'm not sure Darren would have been able to volunteer his agenda when we spoke. The more delicate, embarrassing, momentous or taboo a difficulty is, the less likely someone is to voice it directly. So a patient might make repeated oblique remarks across a number of consultations, subconsciously hoping to prompt their doctor to wonder what they themselves have become increasingly concerned about – for example, that their spouse is developing dementia. Or a young mother, pregnant again, might attend for a string of minor ailments in her first-born, hoping against hope that someone will ask her, out of the blue, if everything's all right at home, because only by having to respond to a trusted person's question will she ever be able to say the words 'he hits me'. In Darren's case, I sincerely doubt he would have been able to phone a doctor and come right out and say his wife was having nothing more to do with their baby and that if he tried to talk to her about it, it provoked a blazing row. Far more acceptable to call about a straightforward medical matter, Harry's food allergies, the thing that seemed to him to have provoked the difficulties.

Peter Tate taught me myriad techniques for drawing out what would not otherwise be spontaneously revealed. There's no pecking order, but first and foremost must be curiosity and care. How is this person being affected by what's going on? And what about those they're in significant relationships with – how are they finding things? When I asked these kinds of questions, it turned the conversation away from Harry and his physical symptoms, and moved it on to Darren and also Lisa. Then there was close listening, both to what was said and unsaid. Asking how Lisa was coping and being told she was out with friends was a non sequitur – the question and the answer were the start and end points of a longer exchange between Darren and me that hadn't been verbalised. Then there were the half-beats of hesitation, and the shifts in speech speed and voice tone, that told me when I was getting onto the right lines.

—

When I studied medicine in the latter half of the 1980s, I was taught to take medical histories – 'clerking' – according to a formula all doctors have used for generations. PC, presenting complaint: what symptoms has the patient noticed? HPC, history of presenting complaint: how long have they being going on, what are their characteristics, how have they changed or evolved? PMH, past medical history: what things have happened to this patient previously and what relevance might they have to what's happening now? DH, drug history: what medications (prescribed, over-the-counter, herbal) are they on; why and for how long? SOH, social and occupational history: what do they do, who do they live with, what is their lifestyle like? Then onwards to O/E, on examination: what the clinical examination revealed.

My daughter, Pippa, now a clinical medical student, has been learning the same formula as I did thirty-five years ago. Only for her there's another section sandwiched between SOH and O/E – ICE. The concept that patients have their own ideas, concerns and expectations is now a standard part of the medical clerking, and has been drummed into her and her contemporaries from their first year. To her it seems like it must have always been there. It's hard to imagine a time when doctors practised without any systematic attempt to understand their patient's health beliefs. When I explained to her that it was my trainer when I was a GP registrar who devised and promulgated the whole concept, she was little short of amazed.

Peter's heart issues saw him leave clinical practice many years ago. *The Doctor's Communication Handbook* is still in print – its eighth edition was published in 2019 – but Peter co-authored its latest iteration with Dr Francesca Frame, an up-and-coming Cambridgeshire GP, because he was aware that he was steadily losing touch with the realities of today's medical frontline. He was awarded an MBE in 2008 for his work on doctor–patient communication. Typical of his self-deprecation, if he mentions it at all he will describe how, after receiving his honour and having a short conversation with the Queen, he moved backwards and tried to turn at the same time, falling over right in front of her.

I didn't know if he appreciated quite how profound has been the change across the whole of medical practice that he set in motion those thirty years ago. So I told him about Pippa's generation of students, and how ICE had become an integral part of the structure of the medical history they are taught to elicit. And I mentioned that every registrar I train arrives in my practice already aware of the concept. I assumed these reports would leave Peter quietly satisfied and proud of his achievements. But he surprised me by being decidedly downcast.

'It's still very patchy,' he said. I was disconcerted to see sadness flit across his face. Peter is an eternal optimist, who invariably greets life's downsides with a broadside of stoic good humour. 'The great mistake was in defining the task,' he said, 'but not the skills needed to do it.'

I knew what he meant. Jim is entirely typical of the registrars I train: he learned the importance of ICE right from his earliest days in medical school, but the way he was taught to approach it (if he was taught at all) was decidedly bald and clumsy. 'What did you think was wrong?' he asked Deepti. Direct and to the point: yes. But her expression and her retort – 'That's why I came to the doctor!' – echoed the bemused or nonplussed reactions I've seen with countless patients when faced by what seems to be a doctor who's out of ideas. Other variations come across just as crassly. If a doctor asks 'What are you worried about?' it all too easily appears they think the problem is trivial and that the patient is overreacting.

These moments in consultations are jarring and embarrassing, and serve to undermine a doctor's apparent competence. Small wonder that eliciting ICE is, for many of the young doctors I work with, an awkward or disliked exercise to be got through as quickly as possible, rather than an opportunity for genuine curiosity and connection. Time and again I see them tick the ICE box then move hurriedly on, metaphorically issuing a sigh of relief that their blunt question didn't seem to have uncovered anything that needed too much attention – and completely oblivious to the undercurrents that remain untapped.

It was something I had subconsciously wanted to gloss over with Peter at our lunch, hoping he wouldn't realise quite what has become of his work. The subtlety and finesse with which he got to know his patients and their agendas – and the affectionate respect in which he held them – haven't propagated alongside his ICE model, which is all too often translated into a transactional, two-dimensional version of what genuine patient-centred consulting should be.

'Back in the eighties,' Peter said, 'I thought it would be done and dusted within my lifetime, that by now everyone would be practising that way.' He looked rueful, sitting across the makeshift table in his garage.

I wanted to cheer him up. 'Sure, but paradigm shifts in medicine take a long time.'

'I don't know, Phil,' he said. 'I think we probably lived through the golden age of patient-centred medicine without realising it wouldn't last.'

—

One of the beauties of general practice is that patients are easy to get hold of if you think you need to review them. At the end of our joint surgery, Jim decided to give Deepti a ring. I pointed out a sign that I'd learned when I was a registrar, that Deepti and Jim had been playing 'consultation tennis'. She'd mentioned fatigue once but Jim hadn't engaged with it – the equivalent of a tennis player returning a serve. So she'd cited fatigue a second time – the consultation equivalent of sending his return back over the net for him to have another try. If someone keeps mentioning the same thing in a consultation they're telling you it's important, and that you haven't dealt with it to their satisfaction as yet. I bet him he'd discover that fatigue would turn out to be integral to Deepti's ICE.

I also talked him through some ways he could more naturally open ICE conversations. He could reflect the 'tennis' back to her – 'I noticed you mentioned fatigue a couple of times. Is that something that's really bothering you?' – and see where it led. Or he could try a more open approach. A simple awareness that patients usually research their symptoms can be really useful. 'Lots of people read about their symptoms online. Have you found anything out?' not only gives a patient a blank canvas to paint on but it tells them you're expecting them to have their own ideas and are interested to hear them. Alternatively, knowing that health matters are frequently discussed at home can provide another non-threatening avenue. 'What do your family or friends think about it all?'

Jim made the call on speakerphone. Deepti was initially surprised to hear from him.

'Nothing to worry about,' he assured her. 'It's just I was thinking back on our conversation and I remembered you mentioning how tired you were feeling. And you said you were still getting night sweats, too. I don't think I ever came back to you about those. I guess I was wondering if you knew anybody else who'd had a similar thing? If it was ringing any kind of bells for you?'

'That's so kind of you, doctor!' Deepti was audibly pleased. 'And you're right. It's my uncle, you see – he was exactly the same, and he had TB.'

'You were wondering if that's what you've got?'

'He stayed with us for three weeks.'

'When was that?'

'Earlier in the summer. Most of June, actually.'

'And he had TB?'

'Not then, no, doctor. That was several years ago. Before Covid, certainly.'

Jim said he was glad to know. He still thought hers was a viral infection that was on its way out, but he could see why she'd been concerned. He offered to ring her back in a fortnight to double-check that it had all got better. 'If for any reason you're not 100%, I can bring you back in.'

'I would really appreciate that, doctor.'

'I'll speak to you then.'

'Thank you. Thank you very much indeed.'

There proved to be no drama. Two weeks later, Deepti was fully better and happy to leave everything there. I know it would definitely have made some difference, the fact her worry had been put out there for Jim to hear and consider. And who knows, he might have averted a repeat appointment, or a 111 call or even a trip to A&E, had Deepti's worries remained unaddressed and gnawing away at her after she'd been in that day.

Things weren't so simple for Lisa. Concerned by what Darren had told me, I spoke to Tracey, the health visitor, and she agreed to go back round. Lisa was in an agitated state, consumed by anxiety and barely sleeping, her thinking overtly irrational. In her mind she was a terrible mother who had nearly killed Harry by feeding him scrambled egg. Tracey got her in with a female colleague of mine whom Lisa knew well (and it was best she had her own GP in case there proved to be interpersonal issues with Darren) and a picture emerged of significant postnatal depression, which she'd been battling against for months on end and managing to conceal from virtually everybody. Harry's second food allergy had brought everything crashing down.

Intensive support and antidepressant medication bore fruit over a two-month period. I shored up Darren, helping him arrange compassionate leave from his job while he got a family rota organised to help look after Harry. Tracey kept a careful eye on the situation, but Harry made it through the crisis the least scathed of the lot of them. When he was eventually assessed at the allergy clinic he proved not to have any problem with egg. What had looked like an allergic reaction must have been a coincident viral gastroenteritis instead. He still has to avoid tomato.

—

When Peter Tate first articulated the ICE concept, the World Wide Web was but a twinkle in creator Tim Berners-Lee's eye. Most patients' experience of medical consultations still conformed to the centuries-old paternalistic model. It generally fell to patient-centred physicians to take the lead in drawing out their patients' perspectives.

Now, Dr Google and the AI revolution have put masses of medical information within anyone's reach. I still encounter a fair amount of reticence among patients about spontaneously revealing ideas, concerns and expectations. But things are changing. Over the past few years, I've been struck by the noticeable minority who begin a consultation by laying their ICE cards on the table. In part this might reflect the way we try to practise in my surgery; patients are becoming ever more used to their doctors wanting to know what their perspectives are. And in part it is a function of the wider cultural changes we're living through.

It feels like we're in a time of transition. In another generation, there may be no need of artful skills on the part of doctors to uncover patients' perspectives. These will be offered as a matter of course, and our chief task will be to negotiate health beliefs informed by widespread but frequently contextless medical information. My hunch is, though, that Peter's contribution to the practice of medicine will always be needed, because there will always be people whose ICE are subconscious or unformed, or feel too daunting to articulate.

Far from having lived through the golden age of patient-centred consultation, I am sure our patients will demand it of us ever increasingly. It's not just about working out what someone's symptoms actually mean. There's the whole issue of obtaining properly informed consent as to whether to take drugs for primary prevention. Or whether or not to be screened. Advances in medical genetics promise to give rise to ever more warnings about conditions we might be prone to, but what, if anything, should we do? The bewildering range of treatment options available as a result of inexorable scientific advance needs to be weighed and tailored to what each individual values. But to practise like this takes time. Assumptions are always quicker than explorations. Instructions are swifter than negotiations. And this is where I believe Peter's gloomy prediction may have some basis.

The Covid pandemic accelerated changes that had been progressively affecting the NHS, and particularly general practice, since the onset of austerity. The sustained real-terms funding squeeze – the longest and deepest in NHS history – has driven workloads and time-pressures relentlessly upwards. GP numbers have been falling since 2015 and repeated government promises to recruit more doctors to the ranks have failed to bear fruit. The average GP is now trying to care for 2,200 patients, a list size that would have been deemed excessive a generation ago, in an era of paternalistic practice and therapeutic simplicity. In today's world of multimorbidity and therapeutic complexity, compounded by the backlog in demand that is manifesting itself as the pandemic recedes, the working day has become about survival. Safe capacity is routinely breached, and more than a third of general practices report having had to close their doors at times as a result. In such an environment, patient-centredness feels like a luxury that cannot be afforded.

Some people worry that changing methods of consultation will also damage the kind of medicine Peter Tate strove to make routine. The UK NHS switched wholesale to a 'telephone first' model during the Covid first wave, and although in-person consulting is gradually recovering, it looks likely that a sizeable proportion of general practice consultations will continue to take place remotely – not least because it is convenient and popular with many patients. In fact, I don't believe remote consulting like this is a barrier to patient-centred communication. My several conversations with Darren took place entirely on the phone, and to this day I have not yet met him face-to-face. It is undoubtedly true that in-person consultations provide rich additional information to both clinician and patient – the majority of human communication is non-verbal and through body language – and I would argue that with any new illness, doctor and patient should be in the same room on at least one occasion. But remote consultation is certainly not an absolute barrier to holistic care.

What is needed is time to practise medicine properly. If the government fails to invest adequately, and fails to direct resources where they are needed, then patient-centred consultations may never become the norm. They will be in the private sector, where adequate time will be funded by those who can afford it. The NHS may be reduced to a transactional safety-net service for those without the resources to exercise choice.

This matters. Patient-centred consulting is much more efficient for the health service, already proven to reduce prescribing costs, and I am certain it would also be shown to be associated with lower activity levels both in general practice and in hospitals. Beyond that, though, it results in far greater patient satisfaction. People feel listened to and understood, and properly involved in their own care. That is healthcare that is genuinely worth having.

9

TAXI-RANK MEDICINE

Red and swollen from mid-shin to below the ankle, something was very wrong with Daniel's leg. It looked like cellulitis, a bacterial infection of the skin and subcutaneous tissues. I regularly cure cases with antibiotic tablets at home, but Daniel's presentation had been unusually rapid and was uncharacteristically painful.

'I think we'd better send you in.'

There was a half-beat of hesitation before he agreed. He and his wife, Lydia, cover the childcare between her work at a nursing home and his maintaining industrial refrigeration units. Anything unanticipated necessitates a rapid ring-round of friends, and sometimes shift cancellations. Daniel didn't question whether hospital admission was necessary, though. I've looked after the family for years, including, at different times, both Lydia and Daniel when their just-about-managing lives have got too much. He knows I wouldn't admit him unless I had to.

In hospital, blood tests seemed to confirm the diagnosis of a severe cellulitis and he was treated with powerful intravenous antibiotics. His leg failed to improve. Scans showed a possible infection in the ankle joint, a complication that would require urgent surgery. The orthopaedic team took over, but an attempt to draw infected fluid out of the joint with a needle proved fruitless and a more detailed scan failed to replicate the original finding. Over the next fortnight, Daniel's leg made limited progress. He was still on crutches when he was discharged with a carrier bag full of antibiotics. I signed him off work; at least he was home again to help Lydia with the daily juggle. I told him I was glad he seemed to be on the mend, even if the diagnosis remained a mystery.

—

Professor Sir Denis Pereira Gray was leaning against the railings outside Exeter St David station when I emerged. He was easy enough to recognise; I'd seen him on Zoom seminars before. It was summer 2021 and Covid was still very much a live issue. We did a cordial elbow-bump then he led me to his small hatchback which, at six feet tall, he had practically to fold himself to get inside.

I don't know if it was on our route or if it required a detour, but he drove me past the building that used to house his practice. He slowed the car as we approached a white-rendered Victorian Gothic revival villa on our left.

'That window there,' he said, pointing to the upper storey. 'That's the room I was born in.'

Pereira Gray comes from a long line of doctors. He eventually took over the practice in which both his father and grandfather before him had been GPs. When he'd been a child, the downstairs had been given over to a waiting area and consulting rooms with the family living above the shop. He and his father extended the building in the 1970s, but by the early 2000s the practice had outgrown even the expanded accommodation. For the past fifteen years the St Leonard's Practice has been housed in modern purpose-built premises sited on the town's former bowling green.

We parked there a few minutes later.

'Right, let's go and introduce you to the others.'

A former president of the Royal College of General Practitioners, and the first family doctor to be elected chair of the Academy of Medical Royal Colleges, Pereira Gray was knighted in 1999 for his contribution to quality and standards in general practice. In 2010 he was voted by his peers to have been one of the most influential GPs of his generation. Although now retired from clinical practice, he continues to lead his research group with the energy and intellectual rigour of someone half his age (he is in his mid-eighties). His two key collaborators are Professor Phil Evans and Dr Kate Sidaway-Lee. Both were in the upstairs conference room waiting to meet me.

Continuity of care – a patient being looked after by the same doctor over a long period – has been the focus of Pereira Gray's research for decades, and his Exeter group are international authorities on the subject. In 2018, the trio were co-authors of a landmark review paper, which looked at all the studies on continuity published worldwide since 1996. They found evidence from numerous different countries and cultures that continuity reduces death rates. The finding was true in both general practice and hospital settings. Continuity of care saves lives.

'And it's not just in medicine,' Pereira Gray explained, once our meeting had got underway. 'It applies equally to midwifery, where continuity reduces perinatal mortality [the death of babies] by 16%.'

Pereira Gray, Sidaway-Lee and Evans took turns to present published research evidence for the myriad other benefits of continuity. Patients are more likely to follow lifestyle advice, attend screening and vaccination appointments, and stick to a course of treatment. In terms of benefits to the NHS, continuity reduces prescribing costs, results in fewer referrals and protects the health service against litigation costs.

'And it doesn't take long to build,' Pereira Gray added. Other studies have shown that patients' relationships with their doctors typically deepen over just eight meetings, while a doctor's sense of responsibility for a patient is heightened after a mere two consultations. These appointments may be over minor complaints, too – a viral infection, a contraception query, a skin concern.

'None of us know when some serious health problem will strike,' Pereira Gray said. 'But the apparently unimportant everyday stuff lays the foundations of the relationship for when it does.'

Continuity of care was once widespread in the NHS. Like most people of my generation, I can still name 'my' doctor – Dr Forshaw – the GP who looked after my family when I was growing up. He had a partner, Dr Critchley, whom one might see during periods of leave, and I recall on one occasion consulting a locum about a knee injury, but other than that Dr Forshaw was the mainstay. Today the picture is very different. The annual *GP Patient Survey* conducted by Ipsos MORI since 2006 has been tracking the proportion of the population who feel they have this kind of relationship with their doctor, and it has been declining every year. In 2021, the figure dropped below 50% for the first time. In 2022, it had nose-dived to just 38%.

A common objection that the Exeter group hears when presenting the evidence of the importance of continuity of care is that it is no longer attainable. Modern practices are ever larger, many now have dozens of GPs serving tens of thousands of patients. The trend towards portfolio careers – where doctors combine work in their practice with external professional roles – and the increasing numbers working less-than-full-time in order to balance work with family life, or to protect from burnout in an increasingly pressured role, mean that fewer GPs are physically present every day of the week. But Pereira Gray's research shows that neither of these need be a barrier. Staffed entirely by less-than-full-time doctors, St Leonard's itself has impressive levels of continuity. And through his networks, Pereira Gray knows of several other very large practices that manage to deliver comparably high, or even higher rates. But he is clear that as practices merge and expand, and as doctors' working patterns change, the default is for continuity to disappear unless deliberate measures are put in place to preserve it.

'General practice is quietly splitting into two factions,' Pereira Gray told me. There are the surgeries for whom continuity remains an important goal, which he places in the minority. The majority of practices seem to regard all doctors as equivalent and provide what he terms 'taxi-rank medicine', each patient contact representing a fresh 'passenger' merely to be picked up by the next available clinician.

At the end of my visit to St Leonard's, I signed the visitors' book. Mine was the first entry after a Covid-enforced gap of eighteen months, but earlier pages were a roll-call of everyone who has come to learn first-hand from Pereira Gray and his research group. They have been highlighting the importance of continuity for years, yet have seen scant attention paid by those responsible for running the NHS, nor from more than a minority of the GP profession. As he told me towards the end of our meeting, 'We've been a lone voice for a very long time.'

—

A couple of weeks after discharge, and while still taking oral antibiotics, Daniel's leg deteriorated. I took urgent bloods, which painted the same picture. I got on the phone to the orthopaedic team. They reviewed him immediately, but still couldn't arrive at a diagnosis. Next stop was an urgent rheumatology appointment, where the consultant ordered a battery of tests. What had looked like a simple if refractory leg infection had become a bewildering maze of rare diagnostic possibilities, some of them potentially life-altering.

The weeks off work turned into months. Daniel's sick pay provision dropped. The family's savings buffer exhausted, Lydia took on extra shifts to keep them afloat. In chronic pain, Daniel sank into depression. We'd been here before, he and I, several years ago, at a time of comparable life difficulty. I prescribed again the antidepressants that had been effective then and referred him for counselling support.

Lydia came to see me, experiencing chest pain and palpitations. A careful evaluation and a listening ear enabled her to understand them not as the heart problem she feared, but as manifestations of the strain she was under. And when Claire, their seven-year-old, began to suffer abdominal pain and nausea, I was able to put it into context – not a 'grumbling appendix', urine infection, nor a life-threatening cancer – but a child reacting to the stresses permeating the family home.

—

Dr Chris Garrett agreed to speak to me for this book on the understanding that I change his name and not identify the large practice where he works. This is one of a new breed that has grown up over the past fifteen to twenty years, the result of government policy to push general practices to work 'at scale', coupled with the 2004 contract that saw the advent of a type of doctor that didn't exist twenty years ago: the salaried GP.

The organisation that employs Garrett is an amalgamation of three smaller surgeries, with close to 30,000 patients. Prior to the merger there were sixteen GP partners working across three practices, and each doctor had a long-term commitment to their surgery and its patients. The new super-practice is run by just four partners, with the vast majority of clinical work done by salaried GPs like Garrett, who have no control over how services are designed and delivered. If they find them intolerable, their only option is to move on.

Garrett is typical of many of his generation. In his mid-thirties, he operates a portfolio career, working two days a week at the practice and another two in his local hospital's stroke service. On Wednesdays, he is involved in a research project looking at falls among the elderly. 'In some respects, you could say I'm part of the problem – another one of those part-time GPs,' he told me. 'But I need to have a balance just to survive.'

He described how comparatively 'civilised' his hospital role is: fixed clinics with adequate appointment lengths and a ceiling on the number of patients, a half-hour lunch break, and a reliable finish time. 'In general practice, I'm working thirteen-hour days, at the end of which I'm just broken.'

When Garrett joined the practice, virtually every ten-minute appointment was reserved for booking on the day, meaning patients were effectively unable to book ahead. The partners had done this in response to government pressure to prioritise swift access. The practice's figures for the proportion of patients dealt with on the same day look, on the face of it, exemplary. But the price that patients pay is the daily 8 a.m. dogfight for an appointment. This can involve an hour or more spent pressing redial to try to get through. When they do, patients frequently find that all the slots are gone. They will have to do it all again the next day.

It's a system that precludes continuity. 'If I want a patient to follow up with me,' Garett explained, 'I have to tell them to ring in on a specific day. Hopefully they'll get through. Hopefully, I'll still have a slot available if they do.' It is such an unreliable system – and one that some patients simply cannot negotiate – that Garrett ends up contacting those he feels most need his ongoing care. These consultations are in addition to his contracted appointments, lengthening an already punishing day.

At one point, Garrett told me, he approached the partners. 'I said, "When did GPs stop seeing continuity of care as integral to what we provide?"' They grudgingly agreed to convert a few of his on-day appointments to follow-up consultations. That helped, Garrett said, but it was nowhere near enough.

Not all his salaried colleagues are as conscientious. Some GPs, Garrett told me, will simply do whatever is necessary to close a consultation within the allotted ten minutes, avoiding engaging thoroughly because they know that next time the patient calls, they are likely to be someone else's problem – what is frequently called the 'collusion of anonymity'. 'There's a lot of variation between what people are doing,' Garrett said. It's not that he blames them. 'There's a lot of firefighting, people just trying to get through that day.'

This experience of primary care will be familiar to many patients of large-scale practices, particularly those who have any degree of complexity to their case – a sense of being fobbed off, and of no one taking ongoing responsibility. As well as being dispiriting and damaging, it is highly inefficient, as Garrett explains: 'People end up having five appointments with a succession of different doctors – where one thorough consultation, maybe twenty minutes long, would have got to grips with it all.'

This new breed of super-surgery is the product of government policy. In theory, working 'at scale' was supposed to deliver cost-savings, though this has never been subsequently demonstrated in real life. But while politically driven, many within the medical profession have colluded. The 'industrial' practice, where clinical work is largely undertaken by salaried (and cheaper) colleagues, has in many instances been lucrative for the handful of partners who own and manage them. To politicians with no background in healthcare – and to doctors willing to don convenient blinkers – it doesn't matter whether a patient sees Dr X or Dr Y, or nurse practitioner A or paramedic B. All they need, surely, is to connect with someone, anyone. Recent evidence has emerged as to the price we're paying. There has proven to be a direct link between practice size and patient experience: the bigger the surgery, the less satisfied patients are with their care. A key factor is the loss of continuity.

In contrast, Bourn Surgery in Cambridgeshire would sit firmly within Pereira Gray's minority that continue to prioritise continuity. The practice operates a personal list system – one where each patient knows which GP is responsible for their care and is encouraged, but not compelled, to consult with them. Francesca Frame, the GP who co-authored the eighth edition of *The Doctor's Communication Handbook* with Peter Tate, became a partner there a few years ago. She'd experienced 'industrial'-style general practice in surgeries like the one Garrett works in. When she came to Bourn Surgery it was an epiphany: 'I thought: this is what I have always envisaged – this is what I've always wanted to do.' She served five years in a salaried role there, ignoring three partnerships in less continuity-orientated practices and holding out till a vacancy arose. Like every other doctor at Bourn Surgery, she works less-than-full-time, maintaining an external role with her Local Medical Committee, a body which advises practices in their dealings with NHS commissioners. Frame and her partners are proof of Pereira Gray's contention that high levels of continuity can still be offered to patients in our modern context. It just takes intention and care.

—

The gabapentin I'd started Daniel on some weeks back was finally kicking in – the drug gradually damps down pain signals in nerves – and his symptoms were at last coming under control.

'Yeah, it's a lot better,' he told me.

His leg was still red but much less florid. He was following orders, using the crutches to take the load off.

'Six months, then we'll see,' he said.

'How do you feel about that?'

'At least I know what's what.'

The rheumatologist had finally arrived at a diagnosis, a rare form of destructive joint disease that usually only affects patients with diabetes, a condition Daniel doesn't have. He needed to keep his weight off the leg for half a year, by which stage the limb would have improved as much as it ever would. After that, another team of orthopaedic surgeons would decide what might help any residual disability.

We sorted a further sick note, this one to facilitate benefits claims. With no prospect that Daniel could return to his former role, his boss had let him go. I talked him through the staged increases in gabapentin dose that I hoped, over the coming weeks, would manage his pain.

'How are things at home?' I asked.

'Yeah, good, thanks.'

He was in noticeably better form. After months of uncertainty, he knew what he had to contend with. His boss's decision had crystallised the family's financial circumstances. Although they weren't great, he could now apply for state support and plan how they were going to manage. The gabapentin must also have been playing its part; continual pain is debilitating. The prospect of respite was at last tangible.

I started to draw the consultation to a close, arranging to

review things in a few weeks. But a thought intruded from nowhere: ask him about depression. It seemed incongruous; it was obvious Daniel was in a better place. I even felt irritated by it. What was the point in prolonging a consultation that had already overrun? But despite the internal tussle, I asked him, 'And you. How are you, in yourself?'

He didn't say, 'I'm fine, thanks, yeah, I'm good.' He didn't say anything. Instead, his eyes flicked down and he stayed like that for an age.

—

Professor Martin Marshall found himself in the media far more than he might have liked over the latter half of 2021. As chair of the RCGP, he gave countless interviews, wrote several articles for newspapers, and appeared before the Commons Health and Social Care Select Committee, all to defend the profession against a sustained assault by newspapers like the *Daily Mail* and *Daily Telegraph* over the difficulty in obtaining face-to-face GP appointments as the Covid pandemic ground on.

In spite of this prolonged spell in an uncomfortably hot spotlight, Marshall was upbeat when I interviewed him by video link in November 2021. I first met him back in 2019, just a month after he'd taken office. Then, a key aim for his three-year term had been to advance understanding among politicians of the pivotal role GPs play in the NHS – what he has dubbed 'relationship-based medicine'. This has much in common with continuity of care, but in addition it emphasises the particular expertise that family doctors have when it comes to interpreting the complex interplay between patients' emotions, psychology, life circumstances and physical health (the biopsychosocial medicine we met earlier in the book).

How would he rate his progress on that score, I asked. Marshall shook his head and gave a wry laugh. Just a few months into his tenure the world had been upended, Covid driving a coach and horses through much of what he had hoped to achieve. No one in government was remotely interested in something so complex, intangible and unmeasurable.

'I think the whole health service has become more transactional, less person-centred,' he told me. 'It's had to be, to even begin to cope. Surgeries that are still providing traditional continuity are very much in the minority, perhaps as few as 10%.'

Pereira Gray would agree with that 10% figure, but ironically the slow-motion collapse of the NHS under the strain of both the pandemic and the backlog it has created might prove to be the catalyst that finally forces this loss of continuity to be addressed. In October 2021, shortly before I interviewed Martin Marshall, the *British Journal of General Practice* published the largest ever study conducted into continuity. Researchers at the University of Bergen had analysed the health records of 4.5 million people – virtually the entire population of Norway – and looked at what patients were deriving from a long-standing relationship with their GP. What they found was little short of astounding.

Patients who'd had the same family doctor for many years were 30% less likely to use out-of-hours services, 30% less likely to be admitted to hospital as an emergency and 25% less likely to die than people registered with their GP for under a year. The Bergen academics employed sophisticated techniques to ensure the substantial differences in health outcomes they found were securely attributable to the length of the doctor–patient relationship. The risk of needing emergency care or dying began to decrease once patients had been with the same doctor for as little as two years, and continued to fall steadily thereafter. This 'dose-response' relationship (in which the more you have of something, the more you benefit) strongly confirms causality. Knowing and being known by your GP really is good for your health.

Rebuilding capacity in general practice will be crucial to restoring the health service – in 2024, extrapolating from the government's own figures, we are short of 8,200 doctors in primary care. But we also need to recover continuity. There are many factors contributing to the unmanageable pressures on ambulance services, A&E departments, 111 and GP out-of-hours services, to say nothing of plummeting public satisfaction with the NHS and our stalling life expectancy, but the Bergen study shows that these are exactly the consequences you would predict from allowing continuity of care to be eroded.

Given the strength of the evidence of the benefits of continuity, it ought to be a high priority for politicians and health service leaders. If continuity were a pharmaceutical product, NICE would be mandating its deployment in every guideline it produces – a 25% reduction in mortality is far greater than virtually any drug that NICE advocates. The Care Quality Commission should be assessing the degree of continuity being achieved as a critical aspect of its inspections of general practices and hospitals. The Department of Health and Social Care should be busily devising policies to incentivise its provision.

None of these things is happening – yet. Jeremy Hunt – a former Health Secretary and for two years chair of the Commons Health and Social Care Select Committee – was the first major politician to grasp its fundamental importance. He updated Pereira Gray's 'taxi-rank' metaphor for the present day, decrying the 'Uberisation' of general practice. Restoring continuity was a key recommendation of his committee's year-long enquiry into the future of general practice when it reported in 2022 (and something Hunt appears to have conveniently forgotten since re-entering government as Chancellor in 2023).

Other politicians quickly caught on. Sajid Javid, one of Hunt's successors as Health Secretary, and Wes Streeting, at time of writing the Labour Shadow Secretary for Health and Social Care, both started to pay lip service to the importance of continuity, though policies to ensure its renaissance have yet to be articulated. The same was true in *At Your Service*, the paper on reforming general practice published by right-wing think tank Policy Exchange in March 2022. But the concept of the prime importance of continuity has at last cut through. Denis Pereira Gray is no longer a lone voice. The challenge for both policy makers and the medical profession is how to resuscitate it.

Martin Marshall expressed concern to me that the increasingly powerful argument for continuity might be interpreted by some as necessitating a return to outdated working practices, when surgeries were run by full-time, mostly male partners. It does not. Pereira Gray's research, and Francesca Frame's lived experience, show that continuity can be delivered by modern practices staffed by portfolio GPs. But the government needs to dispense with the micromanagement of clinical activity and the fetishisation of guidelines. It needs instead to re-create a health service with sufficient GPs with sufficient time and aligned incentives to restore this most powerful aspect of medical practice.

—

I still can't say what prompted me to ask Daniel about depression. When he finally spoke, he haltingly told me how worthless he felt now that his working life was at an end. How he'd been researching methods of suicide, and had stored in his garage the things he would need. No, he hadn't said anything to Lydia. I was the only person he'd told.

In the field of suicide risk assessment, this constituted a huge red flag billowing in the wind. I referred Daniel urgently to the mental health team, who scooped him up the same day. A few months later, a card turned up in my in-tray from Daniel, handwritten in block capitals: 'YOU KNOW I'M NO GOOD AT SAYING THINGS IN WORDS BUT THANK YOU FOR SAVING MY LIFE'.

My belief is that, having known him for years, and having seen him in adversity before, something that I still can't put a finger on had set a warning bell clanging in my subconscious. And, trusting me, he'd felt able to reveal his darkest thoughts.

I don't know how any of Daniel's family would have fared in an 'industrial' surgery, under a taxi-rank system. Lydia with her chest pains and palpitations: an emergency admission perhaps, certainly a cardiology referral. Claire with her abdominal pain and nausea: a surgical admission or a paediatric review. As for Daniel, there must be a strong chance that he wouldn't be alive today.

Daniel is now back in full-time employment, albeit in a more sedentary role, and needs hardly any pain relief for the residual symptoms in his leg. I am currently helping Lydia with symptoms of the menopause. I haven't seen Claire for some time, and I trust she is thriving at school. Without continuity of care I believe their stories would have ended very differently. But there are no counterfactuals in life. We have to be guided by the objective evidence, which when it comes to the importance of continuity of care is now watertight and overwhelming.

10

TOO MUCH MEDICINE

I arranged to meet Julian Treadwell outside the old Radcliffe Infirmary on the Woodstock Road. Much of it was familiar from my time in Oxford in the 1990s and early 2000s. The ornate fountain was still there in the centre of the expansive courtyard in front of the main building, but the sweeping circular driveway where consultants and on-call doctors once parked their cars had been paved to make a pedestrian precinct. The matching pair of Palladian out-patient buildings stood like sentinels to my left but were now conjoined by a striking glazed infill extension, part of Oxford University's redevelopment of the former hospital in 2016 to accommodate its world-leading Nuffield Department of Primary Care Health Sciences.

Julian arrived a few minutes later, looking remarkably fresh-faced considering that, at fifty, he was relatively late to fatherhood and his second child had been born just a couple of months before. He apologised that he couldn't take me inside the department for our interview; this was January 2022 and high rates of Covid as a result of the Omicron variant meant a continuing ban on external visitors to university facilities. He led me instead through the redeveloped Radcliffe Quarter and out onto Walton Street in the heart of Jericho, where we found ourselves a table in the Branca café-bar.

—

Julian fell in love with general practice as a fourth-year medical student. He started studying medicine in 1989, four years after I went to Nottingham, and although the bulk of his training was at King's College Hospital, he had the chance to go to Northern Ireland for his GP placement. For two months he swapped the bustle of London for the village of Keady in County Armagh.

The doctors there worked hard, covering nights and weekends on a 1 in 5 rota on top of their daytime practice, but Julian was struck by how happy they were and the satisfaction they gained from their work. They were intimately woven into the fabric of their community – they were practically considered honorary members of some of the families they served. The strength of the bonds was brought home to Julian by one patient who proudly told him she'd been delivered as a baby by the GP grandfather of the two brothers who were now partners in the self-same surgery.

Julian was struck by the extended roles the doctors performed. Yes, they were physicians, diagnosing and treating illness, but they were far more than that to their patients – acting at different times as counsellors and confessors, witnesses and wise life-guides. It was a picture that would be familiar to anyone reading John Berger's 1967 study of a rural English GP, *A Fortunate Man*. Julian came to think of what he was seeing in Keady in terms of a 'priestly role' – nothing to do with God or religion, but something about the GP as the personification of a secular faith in our society's care for the traumas and health challenges that might affect any individual's life. The experience left a lasting impression and was something Julian aspired to emulate when he came to practise in his own career.

He retained that inspiration throughout his postgraduate training in general practice in Ealing. Peter Tate's work on ICE and person-centred consulting now permeated the GP curriculum, simultaneously an endorsement and a formalisation of the humanistic approach that Julian had witnessed during his student attachment. His GP trainer in London embodied a similar compassionate wisdom in dealing with her patients. He recalls observing her with a distressed woman whose life was being rocked by adversity, providing regular consultations throughout the period of personal trauma. Sometimes there are no easy answers, from either medication or formal psychological therapy. Julian remembers her explanation: that often the most important thing a doctor can do for their patient during a time of crisis is simply to 'hold' them while the storms rage. 'Sometimes what people need above all else is to be listened to and given a metaphorical hug.'

At the same time, Julian was becoming aware of the developments and new thinking that I had been exposed to during my own postgraduate training in Oxford. Midwives he worked with during his obstetrics post told him about the Cochrane Collaboration and its mission to distil and disseminate the latest research. The evidence-based medicine (or EBM) movement set in train by David Sackett was beginning to create far-reaching change. Critical appraisal of scientific papers had been incorporated into the GP training curriculum and was being tested as part of the MRCGP examination, with the aim of equipping future practitioners with the skills to evaluate research first-hand. Julian was enthused by the landmark studies of the era – trials like ISIS-2, which had proved the place of aspirin in treating heart attacks, the 4S study, which had demonstrated the role of statins in the secondary prevention of heart disease, and UKPDS, with its apparently incontrovertible proof of the desirability of tight sugar control in diabetes. Medicine was entering an exciting new phase. Julian emerged at the end of vocational training with twin visions. He would be one of a new breed of next-generation GPs, one whose medical practice, informed by the latest research evidence, delivered the very best scientific healthcare to patients, while simultaneously fulfilling the compassionate, humanistic role of the family doctor.

After a year working in New Zealand and two more spent locuming for practices back in the UK, the opportunity came to realise those ambitions. In 2001, he was appointed as a partner at Combe Down Surgery in Bath. Julian took on the running of a cardiovascular disease prevention clinic at the practice, eager to apply his next-generation expertise in EBM to improving the care of patients with heart disease. But he quickly noticed that a change had occurred over the three footloose years since he'd completed his postgraduate training. This was the era of National Service Frameworks (NSFs), the forerunners of QOF. The practice of EBM had already begun to deviate from Sackett's original vision. Instead of the latest research being used to enhance the clinical expertise of the physician, helping them arrive at care tailored to each individual patient, there was now an imperative to ensure adherence to what was set out in each NSF.

Julian had embarked on partnership just as the guideline culture was beginning to take hold.

Initially, though, things seemed OK. There appeared a persuasive logic to systematically ensuring that patients with established heart disease or diabetes complied with optimum drug regimes to try to protect their future health. Regular auditing enabled him to track the practice's performance and to identify instances where the full range of boxes weren't being ticked. These patients could be recalled for intensive input – encouraged and cajoled to align with what guidelines said they ought to be doing, with treatment being escalated when they fell short of the required targets.

In 2004, QOF superseded the NSFs, and now there were financial rewards to ratchet up the incentives for this behaviour – the ménage à trois, with the state firmly seated in the corner of the consulting room alongside doctor and patient. And periodically thresholds would be adjusted. The levels at which someone should be 'diagnosed' with high blood pressure, or diabetes, or deemed 'at risk' of heart disease were progressively lowered. Ever more healthy people were being turned into patients – caught in the medicalisation merry-go-round, just like Michael in chapter 4 with his 12.14% Qrisk score, or Marta in chapter 3 with her asymptomatic, modestly raised HbA1c.

The pressures and inducements of the guideline culture consumed ever more of Julian's time and energy. And they were frequently anathema to that other vision he had for his role. How could he act as each patient's expert ally, working with their unique circumstances and beliefs to arrive at a shared, personalised approach, when countervailing forces required him to focus on the prescriptive demands of QOF?

Striving to meet the escalating workload involved in trying to be both caring physician-priest and medical risk manager took its toll, and the difficulty in reconciling the often opposing roles created a pervasive dissonance. Julian's experiences were far from unique. In my own practice, ten miles down the road, we took the decision to switch off QOF alerts – the systematic prompts on our computer screens itemising the tasks that needed to be completed in order to meet targets during each consultation: blood tests, weight and blood pressure recorded, smoking status updated, perfunctory depression questionnaire completed, drugs that appeared to have been omitted instituted. We decided that when a patient came for help we wanted to focus on what they needed to talk about, and not to allow external agendas to supervene and dominate the ten-minute appointment as they otherwise did. The financial viability of the practice still demanded we feed the QOF beast, so we allocated protected time for one partner each week to attend to the box-ticking in the background. Up in Southport, it was this burgeoning guideline culture that eventually smothered David Unwin's passion for medicine, leaving him simply doling out prescriptions as though 'completely asleep' and clinging on till the day he would be able to take early retirement. Julian, who was only approaching forty, could see no such escape route.

—

There was a certain symmetry to my meeting with Julian in Oxford in 2022. It was where I'd spent the early years of my career before moving to live and work near Bath. I had decamped there a couple of years after Julian took up his partnership at Combe Down and for a decade we practised in the same patch, bumping into each other from time to time at GP Forum meetings. We were acquaintances, though, and I knew nothing of the circumstances that would see him decide to resign his partnership in 2012.

'They were great people, I'm still friends with them,' he told me over our first coffee in the Branca café. 'And I was earning a good living. On paper it was all really good. But after eight years I was burning out. I dropped my time commitment just to try to cope. That kept me going for a while longer. But eventually I realised: I can't do this for another twenty years. It was an emotionally difficult time. Being a GP was what I'd always wanted to do.'

Word gets around among a medical community and at some point during 2012 I heard that Julian had left Combe Down. The next time I saw him I asked what he'd moved on to. He told me he'd decided to return to locum work and 'see what would happen'. He didn't go into detail about the reasons – he just told me that partnership in the NHS had turned out not to be for him. In truth, he probably couldn't have explained it at the time. He was still somewhat shocked by the disintegration of his dream and was at a loss to understand why it had gone so wrong.

It didn't take long to find out, though – nor to discover 'what would happen' in the next phase of his career.

'It was one of those "The paper that changed your life" moments,' he told me, smiling a little self-consciously over the rim of his cappuccino. Around the time of his resignation from Combe Down, the *British Medical Journal* published a seminal article: 'Preventing overdiagnosis: how to stop harming the healthy'. Written by Australian health scientists Ray Moynihan and Jenny Doust from Bond University, Queensland, together with David Henry from the Institute for Clinical Evaluative Sciences in Toronto, the paper opened with a provocative salvo:

> Medicine's much hailed ability to help the sick is fast being challenged by its propensity to harm the healthy. A burgeoning scientific literature is fuelling public concerns that too many people are being overdosed, overtreated, and overdiagnosed. Screening programmes are detecting early cancers that will never cause symptoms or death, sensitive diagnostic technologies identify 'abnormalities' so tiny they will remain benign, while widening disease definitions mean people at ever lower risks receive permanent medical labels and lifelong treatments that will fail to benefit many of them.

Julian read on, experiencing a dawning epiphany. 'I realised, this is what's been happening to me. And to the system. More and more time spent on mechanistic stuff, monitoring blood test results and processing preventative prescriptions. The difficulties of delivering personalised care – the "priestly stuff" – were enormous. There'd been this massive increase in the volume of transactional, EBM-type care, some of which has value but much of which has very little.' He shook his head, as if still trying to come to terms with a bad memory.

The Moynihan paper, and the realisation there were others who were as disquieted about what was happening to medicine as he was, sent him on a reading spree. 'I got *Overdiagnosed* by Gilbert Welch, Margaret McCartney's *Patient Paradox* and Ben Goldacre's *Bad Pharma*. They were mind-blowing. I read all three in the space of a few months.' He was finding kindred spirits, and for the first time in years his passion and enthusiasm for medicine were rekindled. But he had no idea what to do with it. The authors of those papers and books were eminent academics or high-profile physicians. How could he – a peripatetic and directionless locum GP in the south-west of England – possibly find a role in this energising new territory?

The Moynihan paper contained a tantalising announcement: 2013 would see the first international conference on overdiagnosis. It was to be convened at Dartmouth College in New Hampshire, more than 3,000 miles away. And it was surely intended for the kinds of academics and prominent figures who were thinking and writing about the issue – the movers and opinion-leaders.

'I got in touch with the organisers,' Julian recalled. 'I said: "Is this for normal people, too?"' They told him to book a place and come on over, he would be more than welcome.

—

Julian was the educational speaker at one of our GP Forum meetings in 2013. I was in the audience as he reported back on the Dartmouth conference he'd attended. Overdiagnosis was an entirely new concept to most of us, but it was clear it had tapped concerns in many areas of the globe. The conference organisers had been inundated with submissions and ended up selecting 150 presentations from researchers from multiple countries covering overdiagnosis in virtually every area of medicine, from cancer and cardiovascular disease, through mental health and asthma, to stomach ulceration, dementia, osteoporosis and end-of-life care.

Julian talked us through some of the most dramatic papers. There was the startling epidemic of thyroid cancer in the US and South Korea, numerous tumours being picked up on the CT scans habitually ordered by American and Korean doctors for conditions such as neck pain or cough. The data suggested that the major, disfiguring and dangerous surgery subsequently undergone by these patients was entirely pointless, that these incidental findings would never have progressed to clinical disease. Closer to home there was work that showed screening men without symptoms for prostate cancer with PSA caused more harm than good. Another presentation had demonstrated that treating stage 1 hypertension – the bulk of the cases of high blood pressure that we deal with as GPs – had been carried out for years without any direct evidence of its benefit. We might have been wasting our and our patients' time, and creating an eye-watering drug bill for the NHS to boot.

A number of things coalesced for Julian out in the States. He'd been stunned by a re-analysis of the UK Prospective Diabetes Study – one of the landmark studies that had inspired such enthusiasm for EBM in him when he'd been a GP registrar in Ealing, and the trial upon which the whole edifice of tight blood sugar control that now dominates diabetic care under QOF had been based. The presentation in Dartmouth cast the conclusions originally drawn from the data into substantial doubt. Only one of the three drugs studied, metformin, actually did diabetic patients any meaningful good, and that looked to be via a mechanism unrelated to what it did in terms of sugar control. The whole cult of aggressively lowering HbA1c was essentially a sham. Why, he wondered, was this not understood by every GP in the land? There seemed to him to be two related problems: limited statistical numeracy among the medical community, and a near total lack of access to important information that challenged the prevailing orthodoxy.

While at the Dartmouth conference, he met many of the luminaries of the fledgling overdiagnosis movement, including Ray Moynihan, co-author of the *BMJ* paper that had first caught his attention, as well as Iona Heath and Margaret McCartney, both towering figures in UK general practice. During the course of a conversation with them, he tentatively fleshed out an idea as to what he might be able to do to help rank-and-file clinicians counter the overdiagnosis trend. All three luminaries were encouraging, and urged him to develop his thinking further when he returned to the UK.

—

From being a peripatetic and directionless locum in the south-west, Julian has certainly gone on to make a considerable impact. He co-founded, alongside Margaret McCartney – Glasgow GP, writer and presenter of BBC Radio 4's *Inside Health* – a standing group on overdiagnosis within our professional body, the Royal College of General Practitioners.

'This was the biggest transformational movement in the history of medicine,' Julian recollected over our coffee in the Branca café, 'yet back in 2013 no one in the RCGP was even aware of it.'

The group currently has over 300 members, has undertaken original research, contributed to countless national debates about overdiagnosis, overtreatment and overmedicalisation, and defined a set of five principles against which all RCGP policies should be tested to guard against further compounding the problem. Alongside his college role, Julian worked as an adviser to NICE, helping its then chair, former BMA and RCGP president David Haslam, steer the organisation to mitigate some of the unintended consequences of the guideline culture, particularly when applied to patients with multimorbidity. Other projects with NHS Scotland led Julian into the area of polypharmacy and how to solve the seemingly irresistible trend towards loading ever more drugs on the frail elderly and those with multiple co-morbidities. The answer seemed to be shared decision making (SDM), a marriage between David Sackett's original vision for EBM and Peter Tate's patient-centred consultations, the doctor supplying and contextualising information for the patient, and helping them decide which treatments were worthwhile given their circumstances, values and beliefs – much the sort of thing I was attempting with Michael over the question of statins for primary prevention, and Marta and Matilde with their type 2 diabetes. But while I have some (albeit imperfect) data to share with patients like Michael regarding statins, that is essentially a unique example. For virtually every other treatment I might prescribe, the balance of expected benefits and risks is unknown to me.

This was the realisation Julian had during that Dartmouth conference, the idea of what he might eventually contribute. In this new world of evidence-dictated prescribing, both doctors and patients sorely needed to be able to reach personalised decisions. And no one was providing the information to enable that to happen.

'One problem is that all guidelines look the same. There's nothing to give any idea of their relative importance.' Some interventions, Julian explained, have an appreciable high value: beta blockers in heart failure to prevent sudden death, or blood-thinning drugs in a common heart rhythm disturbance called atrial fibrillation to guard against stroke. The guidelines advocating these interventions are indistinguishable from those specifying treatment of mildly raised blood pressure, or chasing tightly constrained HbA1cs – activities that have scant evidence of real-world benefit.

Julian enrolled for an MSc at the Oxford Nuffield Department of Primary Care Health Sciences in order to further research the problem. By asking a large sample of GPs to rate the outcomes of a range of commonly prescribed treatments he was able to expose the assumptions that underlie day-to-day recommendations, as well as the inaccuracy of the information that, were they to engage in shared decision making, doctors would be supplying to their patients. The results, were they not so important, might be considered darkly comic. Time and again across numerous scenarios, clinicians grossly overestimated the chances of benefit compared with what the clinical trials had actually shown. And just as importantly, they correspondingly underestimated the probability of their treatments causing patients harm. Busy doctors, rapidly scanning NICE guidelines and assimilating the take-home messages, assumed that the treatments being stipulated must unequivocally be good things.

Julian – with ample time to burrow into the detail of the original research – knew how far reality differed from working GPs' assumptions. He was sure that if other doctors, and their patients, had access to the details, 'everyone would have the same revelation I had' and many would question the utility of what the guidelines recommended. But how to present the information in a way that was quickly accessible and readily comprehensible?

—

We'd originally pencilled in an hour for our interview, but the conversation proved far-ranging and stimulating so second coffees followed, accompanied by pastries to keep us going. At one point Julian got on his phone to postpone a scheduled catch-up with a colleague so we could continue our discussion without an endpoint.

He'd brought his laptop and wanted to show me his current project, the idea he'd originally conceived at that Dartmouth conference ten years before, which funding from the National Institute for Health Research was allowing him to pursue now on a DPhil programme at the Nuffield Department at Oxford.

On the face of it, it's deceptively simple. A website that can be made available to every GP via their surgery desktop and through which they can access the evidence of the benefits and risks of a multitude of treatments they might commonly consider recommending. The outputs can be shared in real-time with individual patients, contextualised to their personal characteristics, to form the basis of shared decision making. Underlying it is a mind-boggling amount of work. Data from innumerable trials scrutinised and evaluated, and qualified by commentaries as to which kinds of patients they actually apply to, and what they do and do not show. Headline summaries can be drilled into, to provide more specific detail when required.

I tried out a few scenarios. Julian has worked with talented web designers to make the interface intuitive and easy to use. I found answers aplenty and also the same yawning gaps. Copious information about pharmaceutical approaches, and precious little authoritative information about what lifestyle alterations might contribute – not a failing on Julian's part, but a reflection of the biases inherent in evidence derived through expensive clinical studies, and the difficulty of conducting randomised controlled trials on messy and irreducible measures such as dietary manipulation or the undertaking of exercise.

Whether a stand-alone product as now, or if ultimately integrated into GP computer systems in the same way that imperfect statin data can be accessed from my Qrisk calculator, Julian's website represents an important advance. It is now live (www.GPEvidence.org) but there is still the question of eduction and training, and disseminating awareness of the existence of the resource. Some doctors may need to acquire the skills to deploy it in patient-centred consultations, to say nothing of the NHS affording them the time and opportunity to do so – a wholesale shift in system and professional culture is going to be required. I am left with a strong sense of the enormity of the task Julian has set himself, and both how near and how far he currently is to seeing his vision realised. Of course, were bodies such as NICE required to include estimates of benefit size and potential harms for every recommendation in every guideline they produce – to give doctors and their patients a clear idea of what the actual value might be – then Julian's website would be rendered redundant. As it is, his project represents a significant step in a better direction.

We continued our conversation, exchanging thoughts about the state of the profession and the NHS more widely. I said I was thinking of the NHS in terms of the hull of a boat. How when sleek and pristine, it cuts effortlessly through the water. How each health intervention for which there is some measure of evidence represents a barnacle that adheres to the metal. How no individual barnacle will cause any appreciable drag, so can be clamped in place without apparent implication. Yet the more and more interventions we load – on individual patients to take; on the NHS to provide – each of which seems eminently reasonable when viewed in isolation – the more likely it is you will eventually end up with a barnacle-encrusted hull requiring ever more power and effort simply to keep moving forward.

Julian liked the barnacle analogy, but was less enamoured of my intemperate assertion that we should stop clamping ever more of them on – and should prise off many of the existing ones for good measure. We can't keep loading ever more demands to prevent disease onto the NHS. That belongs in the realm of public health: taxation, regulation, information, advertising controls, addressing socioeconomic deprivation and insecurity – measures that would shift the health of the entire population and prevent far more disease than the NHS ever could in its quest to identify and 'treat' the supposedly higher-risk individual.

How, though, Julian challenged me, to decide what is worth keeping or implementing, and what we would be better off jettisoning or not offering at all? Even more to the point, who should make those decisions? Should it be NICE, with its narrow focus on the cost–benefit of each drug or operation or technology in isolation, with no wide-angle appreciation of cumulative implications to patients or the system? Or individual clinicians like me, with my own biases and beliefs as to what I might deem meaningful? Or do the choices and trade-offs in fact belong to each individual patient, with their unique values and beliefs and circumstances, and who are, after all, the owners of their own health?

—

One of the upsides of the academic path that Julian is currently pursuing is both the need and the time to read widely. In the course of our conversation, he mentioned a couple of references, neither of which I had come across before but both of which I latterly sought out.

One was from the *Journal of the American Medical Association* from 2016. Written by Don Berwick, professor of paediatrics at Harvard and head of the Institute for Healthcare Improvement in Cambridge, Massachusetts, the paper was entitled 'Era 3 for Medicine and Health Care'. Berwick described two earlier epochs in medicine. Era 1 was by a considerable degree the longest, 'with roots millennia deep – back to Hippocrates'. It was characterised by a sense that the profession of medicine is noble, that doctors possess special knowledge that is inaccessible to others, that their practice is beneficent, always seeking to do good, and that they can be trusted to self-regulate.

This idealistic picture was shaken once systematic evaluation of care gathered pace in the latter part of the twentieth century alongside the heady expansion of scientific medicine. Think back to the way only a few units were treating heart attacks as a clotting problem before publication of the ISIS-2 trial. Even more crucial was the quite sizeable minority who remained slow to adapt afterwards in light of the dramatic new evidence. There were scandals such as the high death rates in children's heart surgery at the Bristol Royal Infirmary in the 1980s and early 1990s. These made headline news, but every day in undramatic ways GPs and hospital doctors around the country would be practising to different standards – rarely with conscious negligence, almost always acting in good faith, but nevertheless with unacceptable variation in quality and safety.

These inconsistencies gave birth to Berwick's Era 2, in which guidelines, scrutiny, measurement, rewards, penalties and pay for performance evolved as remedies. In the UK these manifested in first NSFs, then QOF, and more widely across all medical fields as the prescriptive guideline culture. Few would argue that the provision of evidence to inform best practice, and accountability for how well it is offered to patients, is anything other than good. Yet the corrective culture that has arisen in Era 2 has generated its own egregious results. Coinciding as it has with the rise of evidence-based medicine, a seductive fallacy has taken hold: that in virtually any medical scenario there is one size that should be made to fit all. Evidence has come to dictate, not inform, medical practice, its application enforced by targets, financial incentives and punitive regulatory oversight.

Reading Don Berwick's article created for me an epiphany comparable to that which Julian experienced back in 2012 with the Moynihan paper. As I absorbed the implications of Berwick's analysis, I realised: this is what has happened to me. I entered practice in the closing years of Berwick's first era, inspired by notions of what it meant to be a doctor back then. And I have lived and worked through the inexorable evolution of his Era 2. In trying to solve one set of problems, we are now experiencing whole new conundrums. We have traded one unsatisfactory state of affairs for another.

Berwick sets out his vision for a third era. Some of it pertains specifically to the United States, whose healthcare system is very different to the NHS. But he pinpoints crucial remedies that are equally applicable to the UK. A major problem with Era 2 reactions is they focus on process: this is the way the evidence says we ought to be doing things, we will be rewarded or penalised dependent on how well we conform. Leave aside for a moment that the evidence base is highly partial, dominated as it is by pharmaceutical and technological 'solutions' because those are what it profits industry, and to an extent some academics, to generate evidence for. The heart of the problem is that process is not what doctors (or any other healthcare professionals) ultimately want to deliver. And it is not what patients want to be on the receiving end of either.

Berwick touches on the key characteristic of Era 3, and it is what also preoccupies the authors of the other reference Julian gave me, 'Defining Value-Based Healthcare in the NHS', the 2019 report from the Centre for Evidence-Based Medicine at Oxford, the body David Sackett was appointed to as founding leader during my postgraduate training. Value-based healthcare is the idea that just because there is evidence that something can be done, doesn't necessarily mean there is value in doing it.

At the system level, this involves moving away from our current paradigm where bodies such as NICE decide on the cost–benefits of healthcare interventions on an isolated, case-by-case basis. In a context of finite resources, any one activity chosen for implementation is another which cannot be afforded. And thinking back to my boat analogy, any barnacle you choose to clamp on the hull contributes to slowing and drag.

What mix or balance of services and treatments delivers the greatest value – in terms of cost–benefit, yes, but also with regard to other important considerations such as justice and equity? These are important questions to address within the NHS but are also questions for wider society. What represents greater value: to continue to plough money into our health service and expect it to pick up the pieces arising from poor public health? Or to divert resources to address education, nutrition, socioeconomic insecurity, poverty and the lifestyle and environmental factors that generate so much of our modern-day disease?

Important as population value considerations are, as a practising physician I am even more inspired by the other facet of this Era 3 approach to healthcare: personal value. It is the voice of the patient, which has been silenced for so much of medical history. This was, excitingly, beginning to be rectified in the dying days of Era 1 with the work of Peter Tate and others trying to shift the culture towards patient-centred medicine. Era 2, with its relentless focus on conformity to process, has progressively smothered the patient voice again – which is what Peter meant by his gloomy verdict that we have passed the heyday of patient-centred medicine. A new focus on personal value will depend crucially on the style of practice that Peter devoted himself to seeing become the norm. And, as Berwick points out, it has the potential to ameliorate system pressures.

> The more patients and families become empowered, shaping their care, the better that care becomes, and the lower the costs. Clinicians, and those who train them, should learn how to ask less, 'What is the matter with you?' and more, 'What matters to you?'

Era 3 healthcare requires a restoration of trust on the part of government and health service leaders in the intrinsic motivation of almost all of those who work in health to deliver the right care for each of their patients. There would remain a place for oversight and scrutiny but as Berwick argues, the excesses that evolved in Era 2 should be dramatically scaled back and be focused on learning and improvement in patient-reported outcomes, not carrots and sticks with which to drive impersonal processes to conform to a partisan, impersonal evidence base.

—

Julian walked back with me towards the Nuffield Department where he would resume his day's work, and from outside which I would wend my way back through Oxford's city centre towards the park and ride bus and my way back south-west. The movement Julian joined at its inception in 2012 has grown exponentially over the ensuing decade. In 2014, the *BMJ* began a major series of articles under the 'Too Much Medicine' banner, bringing overdiagnosis concepts to a wide audience. The NHS in Scotland and Wales have espoused the key tenets of patient-centredness and value-based choices in their 'Realistic Medicine' and 'Prudent Healthcare' campaigns. NHS England, though beginning to catch up, has been slower to recognise the imperative of focusing healthcare choices at the level of the individual patient. Its attention has been largely concentrated on population values and system improvements, dictating what should be available to patients rather than empowering clinicians to work in partnership to decide what is in each person's particular interests.

On our way through the redeveloped Radcliffe Quarter, I asked Julian if he was still doing any general practice. He used to, he told me, working a day or two a week to keep in contact with the profession. But Covid, and his DPhil, to say nothing of the demands of a young family, had seen that fizzle out. He planned to return in the autumn, though, probably at a similar level while he saw his project through to completion.

The work he's been doing has the potential to provide an invaluable tool for use in the shared decision making that lies at the heart of healthcare based on personal value. Maybe, if Julian achieves his aims, he will have played his part in creating a culture in which he could contentedly return to practice the majority of the time – something he's not ruled out, depending on what happens in academia. If so, it would have to be in an environment where he has the time, information and sanction to meld the twin visions he once had for himself as a next-generation – or perhaps that is an Era 3 – general practitioner. One whose medical practice, informed by the latest research evidence, could offer the very best scientific healthcare to patients, while simultaneously fulfilling the compassionate, humanistic role of the family doctor in assisting them in determining what choices hold the most value to them as unique human beings.

11

TWENTY-FIRST-CENTURY DOCTORS

The train from King's Cross brought me in at the east side of the city, sweeping past Sneinton's rows of red-brick Victorian terraces, burnished by the spring sunshine. In the distance were the old manufactories and warehouses of the Lace Market. In the London Borough of Bexley, where I'd lived my entire childhood, the suburban streets were lined by white-rendered or pebble-dashed 1930s semis. Family holidays had been mostly on the Isle of Wight, the Channel Islands, the Dorset and Devon coasts. A nineteenth-century Midlands industrial cityscape was entirely novel, and deeply romantic, to my parochial eighteen-year-old eye.

When deciding where to apply to medical school I'd drawn two semi-circular lines on the map. One had its radius 100 miles from home: anywhere inside that was too close, so the London hospitals were out. The other was at 200 miles: I still wanted to be able to get back for the weekend if the need or want arose. There was no such thing as a university open day back then. I received a glossy prospectus from each of the medical schools within my geographical zone and pored over them, narrowing down the five I would list on my UCCA application.

Nottingham was the youngest medical school in the country at that point. It had taken its first students just fifteen years before, in 1970. Although it was the new kid on the block, it had gained hugely in popularity and was becoming sought-after. The course was attractively modern. Rather than study the basic sciences like anatomy, physiology, biochemistry and pharmacology in isolation, the curriculum was coordinated. Each term was devoted to one or two body systems – cardiorespiratory, gastrointestinal, musculoskeletal and so on – with the relevant aspects across the basic sciences being interwoven. And the traditional division – two years pre-clinical academic study, followed by three years clinical on the wards – had been broken down. From our first term onwards we would encounter patients, carefully chosen so their conditions related to what we were learning in the lecture theatres, labs and dissecting room.

On top of this, every student, during their third year of study, would undertake research that would lead to a science degree. In most other medical schools, anyone wanting to graduate with a BSc as well as qualifying as a doctor would have to intercalate – extending their course to six years. Around 10% of students did, but the rest kept on the five-year path leading straight to medical qualification. In making a science degree an interim step for all its students, Nottingham was equipping them for what it foresaw would be the landscape of their professional lives: a world ever more rapidly and radically changing as a result of research, in which practitioners would need secure scientific literacy in order to keep up-to-date and thrive.

Just as appealing to me, the university offered the chance to experience the clubs, bars and artistic and cultural life of a thriving metropolis, while being based on a stunningly beautiful campus close to the city centre – a parkland setting with rolling downs and wooded glades, centred on the neoclassical architecture of the Trent and Portland Buildings overlooking the ornamental lake. In those days, UCCA applications had to be filled out in order of preference. To stand any chance of an offer from a popular school you had to place it first, or just possibly second behind somewhere understood to be at the very top of the pecking order. Any lower and your application would go straight in their bin. Nottingham, I'd decided, would be my first choice.

I don't remember much about the interview, other than that one of the three men on the other side of the long table had evidently been tasked with playing bad cop. He asked provocative questions relating to my education and experience, insinuating that my motivations were suspect and that I was a timewaster. They were intended to unsettle and test me under hostile fire. I batted them straight back without flinching.

The only other interview I was called for was at Bristol, the most prestigious and historic of the five schools I'd chosen. Another three men on the far side of another long table. They spent much of the fifteen minutes upbraiding me for my temerity in putting their hallowed institution second – second, what's more, behind an upstart. It was only ever acceptable, they told me, for Bristol to be placed behind Oxford or Cambridge, or just possibly Edinburgh. Their rejection came through shortly afterwards, written confirmation of the dressing-down it seemed they'd summoned me all that way specifically to administer. But their pique didn't matter. A few days earlier, my offer had come through from my first choice. I was going to study medicine at Nottingham.

—

I have two daughters, Pippa and Robyn. I swear I've exerted no deliberate influence, but they have each chosen a path that echoes a different side of my own interests. Robyn is studying English Language and Literature at Magdalen College, Oxford, where Oscar Wilde once roamed the quads. Pippa is a clinical medical student at Barts and The London Hospital School of Medicine and Dentistry. The two formerly independent teaching hospitals merged in 1992 and a few years later were subsumed as a faculty within the college Queen Mary, University of London. Despite ongoing attempts to establish 'QMUL' as the universal brand, both staff and students stubbornly persist in referring to their institution as 'Barts and The London', or, more snappily, simply 'Barts'.

The guerrilla campaign to preserve old identities is understandable given the rich history. The London Hospital became England's first officially recognised medical school in 1785. St Bartholomew's followed suit some sixty years later, though teaching had been going on there ever since the hospital was founded in 1123.

Pippa's journey illustrates the revolution in medical education over the course of the last three decades. Barts – which in my day adhered to the rigid divide between clinical and pre-clinical years, and continued to teach the basic sciences as independent courses – is now radically transformed. Pippa's curriculum is based on the 'systems' approach pioneered in places like Nottingham, but it is delivered in an innovative 'spiral' structure, students layering on more depth and clinical relevance as they revisit each system each year. And while Barts still undertakes teaching through lectures and lab work, it also makes substantial use of an educational methodology that didn't exist in the UK when I was a student: problem-based learning (PBL).

PBL was developed in the 1960s for the medical programme at McMaster University in Canada. It turns the process of learning medicine on its head. Rather than building up knowledge through the study of abstract subjects – anatomy, physiology, pathology and so on – then applying the learning to clinical cases in the later years of the course, students are instead plunged in at the deep end. From their earliest weeks they're confronted by complex patient scenarios which initially bamboozle. Working in small groups, they launch into the literature to find answers to the multiple questions posed. Almost without realising they're doing it, they gain key concepts and understanding across disciplines as diverse as pathophysiology and pharmacology, biochemistry and epidemiology, genetics and haematology, psychology and the social determinants of health.

PBL is now a mainstay in medical education. Most UK courses employ it – some, like Manchester, another once-traditional institution, to an even greater extent than Barts. It surprised to me to discover that Nottingham, so progressive when I applied, is actually now a bit behind the times. The popularity of PBL lies not just in its inherent interest (investigating PBL scenarios was one of Pippa's favourite aspects of her pre-clinical course) but also in the skills it causes students to acquire. PBL is not just book learning, cramming in facts and concepts that will quickly fade from memory if not used. PBL gets aspiring doctors to use literature search and critical appraisal to independently find answers to novel scenarios – the very basis of Sackett's original vision of EBM.

It is not just educational methodology that has changed unrecognisably over the past thirty years. Pippa, whose UCAS application was presented without ranking, was invited for interviews at three of the four medical courses she tried for. At Barts, she did encounter a 'three people on the other side of a long table' scenario, but even then the interviewers sought to probe her thinking and judgement, with discussion about the ethical aspects of a medical case involving a terminally ill child that was in the High Court at the time. Her other interviews were based on the increasingly popular OSCE format – 'objective structured clinical examination'. Candidates progress round as many as ten stations, each manned by different interviewers, the different scenarios testing abilities in communication, empathy, situational judgement and so on. Some medical schools are pioneering the involvement of patients alongside academics and doctors in conducting OSCE interviews, giving the broadest possible perspectives on an applicant's interpersonal attributes.

This change in selection process reflects the movement, led by Peter Tate and others, towards patient-centred medicine in the closing years of the twentieth century. The way future doctors were chosen when I applied – based largely on academic performance, with evidence of some extracurricular sporting or musical achievement and quite possibly familial or school connections to the university – had barely changed for over a century. It was grounded in, and helped perpetuate, the paternalism that characterised Era 1 medicine: picking people able to assimilate the immense academic discipline of clinical medicine and then, once qualified, to practise it on essentially passive patients. Of course there have always been those coming through the ranks able and motivated to deliver patient-centred care (I would like to think I am one) but too often the medical educational machine was turning out intellectually bright but emotionally unintelligent practitioners unfitted for providing healthcare in the modern world. Students entering medical school today must still be academically able – A-levels and the BMAT and UCAT entrance examinations ensure that – but they should also possess the kinds of personal attributes that favour therapeutic relationships in which doctors conduct themselves as expert allies of fellow human beings.

Other developments enhance the chances of this further. In my day, you applied with either three science A-levels or Maths plus two sciences. Other avenues of study were viewed with suspicion – at best indicative of a lack of commitment or focus, at worst a harbinger of degeneracy to come. Pippa took History as a fourth A-level. Medical schools these days are increasingly interested in candidates with non-traditional portfolios, now recognising the value of broader interests and perspectives.

Back in 1985, the almost invariable route – entering medicine straight from sixth form – ensured that most doctors qualified around the ages of twenty-three or twenty-four, heads full of theoretical knowledge but, for the most part, with scant experience of life. No fewer than sixteen graduate-entry programmes have since been established at UK universities, taking mature students with previous careers and enabling them to qualify through an accelerated four-year programme. Among my registrars I've had several who've come to medicine via this route: a former practice manager ('Gamekeeper turned poacher', as she described herself), an erstwhile lab-based immunological scientist and an arts graduate who'd spent several years as a designer with a leading international fashion label. All have brought considerable maturity and life experience to their role, enabling them to connect and empathise with diverse patients that much more readily.

Medical education has also responded to criticisms that it was biased towards white, straight, middle-class entrants, which was certainly true when I applied. The generation now coming through more than mirrors the diversity of ethnic heritage in the UK. Initiatives to widen participation are drawing in more students from socioeconomically deprived backgrounds (though the anomalous halving of maintenance support encountered by all students in their fifth and sixth years is a problem that must be addressed most acutely for those without the prospect of family support). Society's increasing acceptance of differences in sexuality – and to a still-lesser extent gender identity – is also being reflected in the medical world, though I am not suggesting there are not still prejudices to be overcome.

But I worry about this brilliant, vibrant next generation. What world have they been drawn to enter into?

—

Jim, my lanky Northern Irish registrar from chapter 8, was talking me through his cases during a post-surgery debrief.

'This one, no, not very interesting,' he said, clicking straight back out of one set of notes. 'Didn't really need a doctor. Woman with new hypertension, I just gave her amlodipine.'

He went to open the next patient's record, but I got him to stop and go back.

'I know what you're saying,' I told him. 'But.' I scanned Jim's entry, noting the modestly raised blood pressure obtained via a series of home readings, as well as the patient's age and lack of other risk factors.

'Tell you what. For tutorial on Friday can you search out the evidence for treating isolated stage 1 hypertension like that and report back?'

Another day. Gill, a fellow trainer's registrar, arrived early for the out-of-hours shift I was due to supervise her on. She knocked and strode straight in, only to find me finishing off a Zoom interview with David Unwin, the low-carb GP from chapter 3. She issued an apologetic look and backed straight out of the consulting room.

Once David and I had finished, I found her outside in the corridor.

'I'm so sorry!'

I smiled and assured her it wasn't a problem. 'That was David Unwin I was talking to. Have you come across him?'

She hadn't, so I gave her a quick run-down of his work. I wouldn't go as far as to say they reached saucer-size, but her eyes noticeably widened as she learned about the success he was having in helping patients reverse their type 2 diabetes. 'I didn't know that was possible.'

Discussing type 2 diabetes brought us to the question of primary prevention of cardiovascular disease. 'What kind of info do you give patients about statins before you prescribe them?' I asked.

'Well, I tell them they'll help prevent heart attack and stroke.' She looked thoughtful for a second. 'Perhaps I should mention common side effects – muscle aches, that sort of thing – but I probably don't.'

'Leave that aside for a moment. What do you tell them about the expected benefits? About how much they stand to gain?'

Confusion clouded her expression. 'I'm not sure I follow.'

'Have you come across NNTs?'

'Number Needed to Treat? Yes. I don't know what they are for statins.'

'Have a guess.'

'I don't know: five, ten?' She looked acutely uncomfortable to learn the dramatically larger numbers of patients she would have to dose for years on end to stand any chance of averting even one cardiovascular event.

Jim came back to tutorial later in the week and showed me all the evidence he'd found for a real-world benefit from putting his patient on a blood pressure drug like amlodipine. His Word document was essentially a blank screen.

'I don't understand why it's on the guidelines, then,' he said.

We talked through the way evidence gets extrapolated to patient groups never originally studied, how marginal gains in tightly conducted trials fail to translate to the real world we work in, the value-free mission-creep that ever-lowering thresholds creates.

'You said she hadn't really needed a doctor,' I reminded him. 'That's only true once she's reached the point of going on drugs – the nurses will do a brilliant job of looking after her then. But your role – what she needs a doctor for – is upstream of all that. What does her high blood pressure mean? Is it a disease, or is it rather a marker of a need to adjust how she's living? What risks does it actually pose her? What else might she do to improve it, in terms of diet, weight, alcohol, exercise? And if she did contemplate embarking on medication, what downsides might there be? And what might your amlodipine actually offer her – as opposed to what she, and you, might assume?'

Jim was quietly nodding his head. 'I'm going to give her a ring,' he said. 'Go through the whole thing again.'

They're extremely bright, Jim and Gill. Academically they're in the top few per cent. And both were selected for their communication skills, interpersonal warmth and ability to empathise and engage with patients. It's their training that has boxed them into narrow thinking. To pass their exams they're expected to be familiar with and adhere to the NICE guidelines for all common conditions. More complex questions – the cons as well as the pros of screening, the phenomenon of doctor-as-medical-risk-manager, the ever-widening definitions of 'disease' and 'risk', the actual efficacy and side effects of drugs, the health benefits of non-pharmaceutical measures – none of it has been seriously addressed.

Pippa hears a lot about this from her dad at home (undoubtedly too much). I agree with her view: medical school isn't the place for a comprehensive examination of the issues. There's so much to learn first about normality and disease, and about what *can* be done when things go wrong. But we need to introduce key concepts at the earliest stage so that students can critically evaluate what they're being taught.

According to Dr Ellen Fallows, GP and vice-president of the British Society of Lifestyle Medicine (BSLM), this is beginning to happen. She recently set up a Lifestyle Medicine module for medical students at Oxford. 'They are so open to learning about the science behind behaviour change, socio-economic determinants of health and the modifiable risk factors of food, physical activity, sleep, stress, social connection, alcohol, smoking, drugs, technopathology and so on.' At present this is an optional module, as it is at the half-dozen other medical schools that have established similar programmes. In only one, Imperial College, is Lifestyle Medicine currently a component of the core course. Under Fallows's direction, BSLM has introduced a curriculum addressing the harms of 'Too Much Medicine', such as over-diagnosis and overprescribing, and the evidence that the medical profession and the public overestimate the benefits and underestimate the harms of medical interventions. These concepts, too, should be introduced into undergraduate education.

The time to expand the issues – for asking what *should* be done, and the imperative to involve each individual in decisions as far as they wish to be – is during the years of postgraduate training. But so many of my educational colleagues are themselves mired in the guideline culture, and pressganged into uncritical acceptance by the incentives and enforcements of Era 2 healthcare. I challenge every registrar I work with and set them thinking about what it actually means to be a doctor. There are many others like me dotted elsewhere. But exploration of these core aspects of our profession is far from systematic among the formal postgraduate training programmes both in general practice and hospital disciplines. It currently feels like a King Canute situation, like we're trying to turn back an irresistible tide.

—

During the second interview I had with David Unwin he shared a personal insight and invited me to include it in this book. It concerned a type 2 diabetic patient at his practice for whom a colleague had prescribed one of the latest sugar-lowering pills. She developed a rare but well-described side effect that caused her to lose consciousness while driving. She survived the resulting crash with thankfully minor injuries and no one else was involved, but the story might easily have ended tragically.

David showed me a copy of his practice's minor surgery consent form – virtually identical to the one we have at my surgery. We use it to record a patient's informed consent to any operation under local anaesthetic. We might be removing a troublesome cyst or an in-growing toenail. Absolutely nothing hardcore. Yet we detail in writing all the potential complications, no matter how obvious, trivial or unlikely: there will be a scar; the wound might get infected; the problem might recur. Then we get the patient to sign it, to indicate they've been told about, and accept, the terms.

Unwin isn't arguing for a similar level of bureaucracy over the initiation of every drug. But his point is important. Compared with the palaver we put patients through in order to gain their informed consent to a minor surgical procedure done while conscious, we dish out potent pharmaceuticals with barely a cursory word. Most patients who experience side effects will get only minor ones. They'll discontinue the tablet, shrug their shoulders, and move on. But the small minority who suffer a far more serious consequence would justifiably feel that they'd been inadequately advised. Informed consent is a basic tenet of all aspects of medical practice, and in matters related to surgery it is generally done well. When it comes to our prescription of drugs, genuinely informed consent hardly ever happens at all.

—

The transformations in medical education when I compare my student experiences with Pippa's feel like the ponderous course changes one imagines with an ocean liner. Pioneers like Peter Tate driving a revolution in patient-centredness, and David Sackett bringing the latest evidence to inform decisions in the consulting room or at the bedside, helped usher in a whole new culture in medicine. They turned the ship's wheel.

The medical educational establishment gradually changed direction in response, seeking to draw in individuals best-suited to what the profession had become, and equipping them with the skills they would need to fulfil their role. Yet the destination towards which their graduates are sailing is currently very different from that created by the work of people like Sackett and Tate. Instead, new graduates find themselves plunged into the heart of Berwick's Era 2, with its rigid guideline culture, polypharmaceutical predominance, trammelling incentives and penalties – a world of cookbook healthcare, patient disinformation and professional dis-ease.

These are stormy, not tranquil, seas. The overdiagnosis movement seeks to reverse the damaging aspects of Too Much Medicine – rescuing Sackett's EBM legacy from the evidence-dictated machine it has become. Integral to that mission is the espousal of shared decision making – offspring of Tate's patient-centred consulting: the involvement of each individual in choices arising in relation to their health, choices the consent to which should be truly informed.

How these countervailing forces will play out will determine the character and shape of Era 3 medicine in the UK. If patient-centredness and clinical autonomy can be restored to the profession, then those we have enrolled to be our replacements will enjoy satisfying and meaningful careers, and will serve their patients – all of us – well. But if we fail to undo the damaging aspects of Era 2, I foresee only more disaffection. Highly intelligent and able people want roles in which they can exercise their talents and skills. If they find themselves trapped in environments that stifle their aspirations to deliver bespoke patient-centred care – the very mission we recruited and trained them for – they will walk away in ever greater numbers than they already are. Who will be left to look after us then?

—

Alfie's world was falling apart. Just ten weeks into his first placement on his postgraduate GP training programme – a six-month block in A&E – he'd been thrown out. His clinical supervisors in the frenetic emergency department had quickly realised he wasn't competent to be allowed to assess patients independently. They'd tried to put support in place, but the level of supervision required to ensure patient safety had been too onerous. They simply couldn't devote that level of resource alongside everything else the substantive doctors had on their plates. Alfie had to go. The deanery asked me, as his educational supervisor, to take him in at my practice until they could figure out what to do.

We'd swapped introductory emails at the commencement of his programme, at which point he'd assured me that all was well, but he hadn't yet taken up my invitation to come out to my practice. This was the first time we'd met. Lean, with the frame of a long-distance runner, he managed a warm smile of greeting, but he must have been feeling deeply disturbed by how things were turning out. I took him upstairs to the coffee room so we could have an informal chat away from everyone else. It didn't take long to get a sense of what had gone wrong.

'I'd never even seen an ECG before coming here,' he told me. Heart tracings are done as standard on numerous UK A&E patients. 'In my country, there's almost no heart disease. Average life expectancy is fifty-five! An ECG would be like referring for a CT scan. The patient would wait months to see a cardiologist in the city, who'd send me a report on the trace. I've never interpreted one in my life!'

There was a forcefulness to his voice that spoke to me of the threat he must feel under. Alfie trained and practised for nearly ten years in his native Africa (I'm not naming the country, and he has been given a pseudonym) before being attracted by the NHS's drive to recruit doctors from overseas. Weary of the corruption and violence endemic at home, the idea of a new life in England was tempting. After extensive family consultation, he'd uprooted his wife and three sons and come over.

The more we talked, the more I appreciated the enormity of the challenge he was facing. The case mix he'd been used to managing was totally different. Infections and tropical diseases, many of which I'd heard of but none, except malaria, had I ever encountered. Malnutrition states I'd only ever read about. Children near death's door from dehydration from simple diarrhoeal illness. Complications of childbirth one would simply never see in the UK.

As for Alfie, he'd never been faced with the kinds of conditions that are the staples of practice here. Yes, he saw cancer, but on the whole people rarely survived to an age at which they might develop the degenerative heart, lung, joint and brain diseases we routinely deal with. 'We just don't have dementia,' he told me. He laughed disbelievingly. 'I mean, sometimes a very old woman might get possessed of evil spirits and wander off into the bush never to be seen again. But that's it!' Overdoses were entirely alien. The concept of child protection – at the forefront of everyone's minds when assessing young patients in the NHS – was similarly new. I tried to imagine how I would cope, getting off a plane and going to work in a clinic in his home town. I doubted I'd last an hour.

Alfie stayed at the practice for the rest of his first six-month block and we set about filling in some of the many gaps in his knowledge base. He was dedicated, turning in a couple of hours of private study every evening to try to bring himself up to speed. Depression was a whole new concept, but he rapidly assimilated a framework for diagnosis and treatment. Although the medical culture he'd been used to was highly paternalistic, he embraced the concept of patient-centred consulting and shared decision making enthusiastically. He did a huge amount of work learning to interpret ECG traces, and devised a teaching session which he delivered to a group of other international medical graduates who, like him, had little experience of the investigation before coming to the UK.

When he returned to hospital placements, the deanery having connected him with extensive professional support and mentoring, things initially went well. He completed a cardiology post satisfactorily, though his supervisor noted his lack of experience relative to his UK-trained peers. But as he rotated to other departments, lapses began to occur. Late arrivals for shifts. A patient not reviewed as per consultant instructions. A fluid regime not prescribed for a critically unwell woman, with serious consequences. Team members complaining that he never put himself forward to take on extra work, and that tasks Alfie had sworn he'd completed often proved not to have been done. For the second time, he was ejected from a hospital training post and landed back with me.

While superficially it appeared he simply wasn't up to the challenge he'd set himself, there were deeper layers. The sheer complexity of many patients was unlike anything he'd previously encountered in his own country. Despite all the book learning he was undertaking, he was struggling to translate the kind of single-disease medicine he was familiar with to the multimorbidity so common in the UK today. There were other buried cultural barriers, too. The strict hierarchies in which he had formerly worked meant it would be impertinent and interfering for a junior to take work from a colleague. Every day was a living nightmare: feeling constantly out of his depth, and aware of his team members' dim view of him.

I encouraged him to see his own GP, and the deanery arranged counselling and a short period of sick leave. Gradually, it dawned on Alfie that his lapses of concentration and frayed timekeeping were the overt signs of the turmoil within. Translocated from all that had been familiar, landed in a world simultaneously overwhelmingly taxing and increasingly hostile, Alfie had developed depression. 'I wasn't even aware I *had* a mental health,' he told me later, managing to laugh at his lack of insight, 'let alone that I needed to look after it.'

Alfie's original three-year training programme has been twice extended, and will now run for an additional eighteen months. He's had to apply for visa extensions for his entire family, at a cost of several thousand pounds. With increased support he continues to make progress, albeit slowly, and he is still practising at a level below where he needs to be.

—

The UK has, for many years, failed to plan for the healthcare workforce it needs. Although medical school places have been expanded, and several new schools established, we continue to train far fewer doctors than we need. The inadequate pipeline is being compounded by the crisis in retention. Older doctors are retiring early in droves, partly in response to intolerable workloads, partly disillusioned by the suffocating constraints they've experienced as Berwick's Era 2 tightened its grip. Other colleagues in mid-career, particularly in the disintegrating world of general practice, are reducing their time commitments and taking on other roles in order to protect themselves from burnout. Young doctors, eyeing the landscape with a jaundiced eye and with the early-life flexibility to swerve in new directions, are moving abroad or choosing to switch to different careers entirely.

In an effort to fill the huge workforce gaps these trends are creating, the UK has increasingly relied on overseas recruitment. The crisis predates the pandemic: numbers of overseas-trained doctors coming to work in the NHS have been accelerating hugely every year since 2016. In 2019, registrations of international medical graduates (IMGs) with the General Medical Council exceeded for the first time those of UK-trained doctors coming on stream.

Alfie's story is far from unique. Two of his contemporaries have quit and returned to their home countries. A third has taken a year out of training to try to consolidate his experience. Until very recently, we have simply dropped these new entrants into training programmes designed for doctors already thoroughly immersed in the NHS and the kinds of case mix and practice particular to the UK. The struggles many IMGs have faced are, like Alfie's story, forcing a rethink. It's difficult to overstate quite how much unconscious knowledge UK-trained doctors acquire through their years at medical school and during their first years of foundation training. The concept of the 'NHS-naive' colleague is gaining widespread acceptance, as are the extended, tailored training programmes they will require in order to be successfully assimilated.

There is a moral dimension rarely discussed: the majority of overseas recruits come, like Alfie, from poorer countries themselves grotesquely short of doctors. In anything but the short-term emergency we have created for ourselves, we cannot go on leaching medical personnel from other nations that can ill afford to lose them. There is an urgent need both to train sufficient of our own citizens and, equally importantly, to carry out wholesale reform of the health service so that it is once again an environment in which people can be retained.

Meanwhile, increasingly dependent as we currently are on the services of colleagues from other countries, we must provide them with appropriately geared training to induct, support and equip them during what are often profoundly disorientating and sometimes alienating personal and professional transitions to practice in the UK.

Part Four

TWENTY-FIRST-CENTURY NHS

12

IN WITH THE NEW

I no longer recall her name, but I clearly remember picking up her notes. They were contained in one of those iconic buff Lloyd George envelopes ubiquitous in British general practice in the 1990s. The white sticker bore her name, date of birth, address and phone number. She was a similar age to me, in her early thirties. And below all that, printed in bold type, the name of her doctor: Dr P.J. Whitaker.

I felt a distinct tightening in my stomach. I'd been building up to this day for months, the moment when I would become a fully-fledged GP principal. I'd qualified ten years before and had subsequently gained a good amount of experience both in hospital medicine and general practice. But although I'd always taken very seriously my duty of care, every patient I'd looked after had been someone else's ultimate responsibility – be that the consultant whose firm I was working for, or the GP principal whose locum I was undertaking.

Now, on my first day as a GP partner, the medical care of this woman whose notes I was holding – the first patient I was due to consult in my new capacity – was going to be down to me. Anything might befall her over the course of her life: inflammatory arthritis, difficulty conceiving a child, scares over a lump found in a breast, depression resulting from an abusive relationship, a disfiguring skin condition, torrid anxiety complicating the menopause. And whatever she faced, I would be the one to whom she would turn. It would be me she would rely on to diagnose and treat her to the best of my ability, and to organise timely additional help if that was what was required. And what was true of that one woman – someone at a very similar life stage to me – was also true of another 1,800 people of varying ages and backgrounds, from tiny newborns to frail nonagenarians, drug addicts to distinguished academics. My list of patients.

Seeing my name on that set of notes crystallised the weight of it. I remember how daunted I suddenly felt. Who did I think I was, believing I could be that person to all these unknown people? Their doctor. It was the huge responsibility of so many other human beings relying on me for so many important and often life-changing things. Could I really be worthy of the trust they would place in me?

I suppressed the sudden wave of apprehension, summoning memories of Dr Forshaw, our family doctor throughout my childhood, and Dr White, who had assumed that role when my parents moved house when I was eighteen. I'd seen first-hand the importance of those long-standing, personal doctor–patient relationships to my dad, whose mental and physical health continued to be affected by his cancer diagnosis and the late side effects of radiotherapy treatment.

I had my role models. Now I had my chance to emulate them. Back then, virtually all GPs were partners in their practice – prior to the 2004 contract the NHS both required and incentivised it. Practices were stable entities, a home for as long as one would want, and when the time came to retire or leave there would be, without question, new entrants vying to take one's place. Indeed, partnership was so desirable that it was common for new incumbents to work for up to five years on a reduced share of earnings. I had negotiated favourable terms – it was only going to take me two years to reach full parity. My future was assured.

—

Marion looked highly anxious. It was hardly surprising. The symptoms she'd been describing, in a woman in her mid-sixties – pain in her mid-back, nausea, appetite suppressed, weight down, a little bit breathless – immediately raised the spectre of cancer. It was now some twenty years since I first became a GP principal. I'd left my Oxford practice and moved south-west, spending three years in salaried posts before finding and joining the partnership where I still work. Along the way I'd gained a wealth of further experience. Listening to Marion, the diagnostic possibilities flicked effortlessly through my mind – cancer of the stomach, oesophagus, perhaps pancreas or lung, maybe spread from an occult breast tumour, or ovarian, or some kind of blood cell malignancy.

There were less sinister possibilities as well: peptic ulcer, medication side effects, liver problems. Investigative strategies formed: bloods first, maybe a chest X-ray, with an ultrasound or gastroscopy to follow depending on the results.

But I'd also known Marion for ten years by then. I carried memories of other encounters we'd had in the past, with similar symptom patterns. While I examined her on my couch, I gently teased out her concern. It turned out to be pancreatic cancer: she'd been researching online and her symptoms fitted exactly. I palpated her abdomen. No doubt she'd also read that tumours of the pancreas are impossible to detect clinically, that they have to be diagnosed by some form of investigation.

Examination over, I sat her back beside my desk and put a reassuring hand on her arm.

'Listen,' I said. 'I think this is going to be fine.'

She looked startled and shifted in the chair. Her voice when she spoke was almost pleading.

'Can't you even arrange a scan?'

She was absolutely right, of course, what she was experiencing could very easily be a textbook case of pancreatic cancer. I had to make a conscious effort to quell my own niggling uncertainty and keep my focus on what I knew was truly wrong. I shook my head and gave her my most confident smile.

'No, no scan. I'm sure this is going to be fine.'

—

Another day, another morning surgery. Ellen brought Charlie in, hoisted up on her hip.

'He seems unsteady somehow. I'm not really sure what's wrong.'

At first glance, her two-year-old looked well. He was reluctant to get down and walk but a lot of young children are scared at the doctor's. I tried him with various toys. In the end, Ollie the Wobbly Owl proved too tempting. Charlie wriggled out of Ellen's arms and toddled across the room to where the clockwork plastic bird was swaying mechanically from side to side. Sure enough, Charlie seemed to have a limp.

The likeliest cause was an irritable hip, a short-lived joint effusion common in kids of his age. But I was aware of a faint unease. The gait disturbance didn't seem quite right. And there was no history of a cold or flu, which precipitate a lot of irritable hips. I wiggled his leg through the full range movement once he was back on Ellen's lap and he didn't seem to mind.

'I think we'd better send him up for a Paeds opinion,' I told her.

She took the news calmly, correctly reading my better-safe-than-sorry tone. Nevertheless, as she was gathering her things, she asked if I thought there was something serious going on.

I shook my head and gave a reassuring smile. 'I don't think so, no. I'm sure it'll turn out to be fine.'

—

The rumbles, when they reached my ears, seemed distant at first. In 2016, I started to hear reports of GP surgeries closing in far-flung places – Folkestone, Swindon, North Wales, Tyneside. The downward spiral was similar wherever the stories originated. One or two partners would leave. This might be because of natural retirement, or they might have decided to go early, burned-out and disillusioned for reasons that, like with Julian Treadwell and David Unwin, they might not have been able to name. Their practice would get no response to recruitment adverts, and workload would pile up on the remaining doctors. The cracks would deepen – a GP out through long-term sickness, another reducing hours in an effort to cope, yet another resigning due to stress. What had once been a healthy, viable, five- or six-partner surgery would be down to one or two remaining doctors, propped up, if they were able to find them, by expensive locums or transient salaried GPs. In the end, the exhausted survivors would have no choice but to hand their contract back and shut the practice down.

Each individual closure causes a domino effect. Thousands of doctorless patients are suddenly added to the lists of neighbouring surgeries (often some distance away), increasing pressure and causing the same cracks to appear in some of those practices too. Brighton and Hove, for example, lost a quarter of its thirty-six surgeries in the space of just four years from 2015. Nationally, over 800 practices have shut since 2013, displacing an estimated 2.5 million patients.

I am fortunate to work in a sought-after part of south-west England; recruitment has never before been a problem. Yet a friend ten miles down the road in the next county is now one of only two remaining in what was once a thriving six-doctor practice. They've introduced a 'last man standing' clause into their partnership agreement, so that neither of them can jump ship and leave the other bearing the costs of staff redundancy and potential premises losses alone. Three of my neighbouring practices, all excellent members of our nine-surgery primary care network (PCN), are currently unable to replace doctors. Two have closed their lists to new patients – an emergency measure to try to stabilise their situations. I see some of the partners on Microsoft Teams, the time-efficient pandemic-inspired way our PCN conducts its monthly meetings these days. They remain outwardly cheerful, but the strain shows in their eyes. All of us are wondering: how long will they be able to go on?

The career that, when I started, was a stable, sure and satisfying prospect, is in slow-motion collapse. And what were distant rumbles just a few years ago have become up-close and personal.

—

Marion returned three weeks later as arranged.

'It's just as bad,' she told me.

I was a little disconcerted. 'The tablets haven't helped at all?'

She looked at her lap, where her fingers were repetitively intertwining. 'I didn't take them. I looked at the leaflet and I saw that thing about them making you go jaundiced, and all I could think about was me turning yellow.

'My weight's gone down some more.' She met my eyes. 'You don't think I should have that scan?'

I took a deep breath and explained about lists of side effects: how, when we read them, it can feel as though every single thing detailed there is bound to happen to us. But that in reality, serious unwanted effects like the liver damage she had fixed on were vanishingly rare.

'I've prescribed them to hundreds of patients over the years,' I told her. 'I've never had anyone have a reaction like that.'

She remained unconvinced. She was certain she had pancreatic cancer. It was frightening that her doctor simply didn't seem to get it. The temptation to arrange a scan was incredibly strong; it would come back normal and give her peace of mind. Yet it would be precisely the wrong thing to do. The relief of anxiety that comes from negative testing is as powerful a drug as Valium, and patients with health anxiety quickly become addicted. Costs to the NHS spiral. Even more important is the risk of causing her inadvertent harm – through radiation exposure, or through the incidental, uncertain findings that turn up on approximately a quarter of tests and which can take many months – sometimes years – of repeated investigations to be ultimately proven to be harmless.

I reminded her of the deal we'd struck some years before. How I promised to take seriously any symptom she developed, and how I would investigate anything that I felt ought to be checked out. But how in return she was to trust me. I scrolled back through her notes with her, seeking out contemporaneous records of past occasions when we'd dealt with similar episodes, all of which had proved to be self-limiting.

'I'll be keeping a careful eye on you,' I told her. 'If things aren't working out as I anticipate, I promise we'll re-evaluate. OK?'

She held my gaze. Her face softened. She gave a nod. 'OK.'

'And do try the tablets. Please,' I said. 'I promise you, you won't turn yellow.'

Ridiculous thoughts kept popping into my mind. How she'd be bound to get liver damage now I'd said that. Or quite how I was going to feel when, after a couple months of no progress, I would finally organise a CT scan which would reveal an advanced pancreatic tumour. But I suppressed the superstitions.

'Come and see me in another three weeks,' I said. 'I'm sure you'll be picking up by then.'

—

Ellen came to tell me she was pregnant.

It was not a surprise; I'd been receiving periodic letters from the specialist centre where she'd been having cycles of IVF coupled with pre-implantation genetic diagnosis. Nevertheless, I was careful not to issue hasty congratulations. 'How are you feeling about it?'

'I just feel numb,' she said. 'I only did it for Ed.'

We sat in silence for a few moments. I weighed things in my mind. The awful days during which it had become apparent that Charlie's limp was the result of an aggressive tumour on his spine. The endless trauma Ellen had been through as her precious boy suffered fear and the terrible side effects of chemotherapy. The desperate hope that it might achieve a cure. The trip, squeezed between treatment regimes, to Disneyland Paris, to give him a fleeting experience of magic. The soul-destruction when, after more than a year of battling, he had finally died.

For the next two years Ellen had seen me virtually every fortnight, sometimes even more frequently. Her notes contained innumerable entries charting the depths of her despair. The engulfing guilt at failing Charlie somehow, compounded by the devastating results from genetic testing – completely unbeknownst to Ellen, she had passed a fatal cancer-causing mutation to him. The unbearable pain of his loss. How despite high-dose antidepressants she had been suicidal for months on end, feeling there was nothing worth living for. She'd hated seeing the psychiatric team, hated talking to strangers who had never known her little boy. They'd found it impossible to help her. I would get periodic distress calls from the childhood cancer nurses, still supporting

Ellen in her bereavement, unnerved by and unable to handle her talk of ending her life.

Somehow I'd contained it, hearing her true feelings and not trying to fix them. We'd gone into uncharted territory professionally. She'd been to a medium, and gradually we evolved a way of talking about Charlie being in another place, waiting for her. She visited his grave obsessively. Sometimes she couldn't see the point of carrying on just to delay being with her son again.

Painfully, slowly, time had started to heal, and she had improved to a degree. And then she'd been offered pre-implantation diagnosis so that any subsequent embryo could be screened clear of the malign mutation before becoming established as a viable pregnancy.

'I've got to go through with it,' she told me, indicating her tummy where a new life was underway. 'But I don't want it.' She shook her head vehemently. 'As soon as it's born I'm going to hand it to Ed. It's him who wants another one.'

Throughout the ensuing months, Ellen would talk about how she felt absolutely nothing for the baby inside her, and how utterly horrible she felt about herself, betraying Charlie by having conceived again – and having conceived a child free of the gene that had killed him. She couldn't express these feelings to anyone – not to Ed, or her family, or friends. Everyone was delighted about the pregnancy, they felt it marked a new, positive, healing chapter. Ellen put on an act for them. Only behind the closed door of my consulting room could she be true to herself.

With Ellen's consent I liaised with Laura, the midwife who had seen her through her pregnancy with Charlie. We carefully considered referrals to child protection and specialist mental health. But we knew how intolerable and intrusive Ellen would find the involvement of outsiders, and we were sure it would make things far worse. Her feelings were very troubling, but referring her against her wishes to other agencies would involve breaching the trust she had placed in us. She would become caught in a well-intentioned but control-sapping whirlwind of procedures and protocols that would quite possibly break her.

Laura and I decided to monitor her weekly between us. We both felt that if Ellen could just get through, then the moment she met her new child the world could change. Laura undertook to ensure that when Ellen came to deliver, she would be the midwife to attend her throughout the labour.

It was a calculated risk, and we would face criticism were things to go wrong. But we both believed, knowing Ellen as we did, that it would prove to have been the right thing to do.

—

Most commentary about the current state of the NHS focuses on chronic underfunding. There is truth in this. The health service in the second half of the 2000s was the best I've experienced during the entirety of my career. Access to general practice was excellent, and where investigations or specialist care were required, they were delivered within weeks. This was the direct result of the governments of Tony Blair and Gordon Brown increasing per capita funding to match that of comparable developed nations. The surest illustration of New Labour's success was the response of the private medical insurance industry. Alarmed by falling customer numbers – why pay for healthcare when public services are so good? – they began to launch cheaper insurance policies designed to kick in only if the NHS failed to deliver on its swift timescale guarantees.

The sustained real-terms funding squeeze by successive Conservative-led administrations since 2010 has wrecked that legacy. Strip out the huge sums recently deployed in tackling the Covid pandemic – much of which was squandered on ineffective contracts with private outsourcing companies rather than invested in established public services – and we are again spending far less per capita on healthcare than most similar countries. Hoardings around sports grounds, adverts on pharmacy front doors and Tube trains hawk fee-for-consultation GP services and medical insurance products. Those with the resources to escape what the NHS has become (and fortunate enough not to have the kinds of health needs the private sector won't cover) are voting with their feet.

Yet increased NHS funding alone will not solve our current crisis. This book has told a series of stories – about movements in medicine, political interference, and social and cultural change – that have interacted in unanticipated and unpredictable ways to alter the role of doctor over the course of my career. Those stories also contain the answers as to how the NHS can be rendered fit to serve the nation's health for the next seventy-five years. The remedies are of equal importance and must be enacted in parallel, but I will describe them sequentially here. They boil down to four Rs.

The first R is to re-professionalise medicine. New Labour may have delivered first-world levels of funding but, with their addiction to centralised control, they firmly embedded the guideline culture through the twin arms of NICE and QOF. We have seen how partial and incomplete the evidence base actually is, serving corporate interests and allowing government to abdicate responsibility for public health in favour of population-level pharmaceutical and technological 'solutions'. Doctors should be delivering care personalised to each individual patient, explaining and taking account of what the best available evidence shows and, crucially, does not show. We need to recover David Sackett's original vision of evidence-informed medicine, and dump the evidence-dictated monster it has become. Governments must step back outside the consulting room, quietly closing the door behind them. We need an end to the ménage à trois.

At the same time, my profession has to face its own culpability. The evidence for the importance of continuity of care – to patients, doctors and the wider NHS – is indisputable. GP partners who have presided over the evolution of 'taxi-rank' or 'industrial' medicine, often profiting personally, must deploy readily available and proven tools to restore continuity of care to their patients. Consultants and managers responsible for hospital departments must do likewise: continuity counts in all medical settings. And medical education must foster a far more critical appraisal of guidelines, not merely training practitioners to apply them slavishly. These measures are within my profession's gift, though they will be greatly enhanced by government policies that encourage and incentivise the restoration of continuity, and patient-centred care. The evidence now clearly demonstrates the folly of policies that have driven GPs to operate at ever larger scale: the bigger the practice, the lower the satisfaction of their patients with the care provided. When it comes to primary medical care, smaller is unarguably better.

Alongside re-professionalising medicine is the second R: rebalancing specialism with generalism. Over the past decade, hospital medicine has undergone rapid expansion – doctor numbers have swelled by more than a third. In part this is due to increasing sub-specialisation, itself necessitated by the breathtaking explosion in scientific progress. We live in a world where the genetic underpinnings of Charlie's tumour can be delineated, where IVF and pre-implantation diagnosis can ensure Ellen and Ed can have a future healthy child. A world where, were Marion to prove to have pancreatic cancer, she would be cared for by a surgeon who spends their days planning and performing operations on just this one part of the body. Where oncologists could offer her chemotherapy and immunotherapy tailored towards her specific disease.

This trend towards sub-specialisation is highly beneficial: patients with serious conditions get the best care from professionals who concentrate exclusively on their particular problem. They will be highly skilled at its management and in performing relevant technical tasks. Yet while specialist numbers have burgeoned, there has been a corresponding decline in doctors in general practice. Numbers flatlined for years and since 2015 have been falling steadily, currently down by nearly a tenth. This matters. For every child like Charlie who I send for specialist care, there are dozens and dozens who go nowhere near a hospital because I safely manage their illnesses in the community. Were I to refer everyone like Marion, whose symptoms suggest pancreatic cancer, my gastroenterology colleagues would be rapidly overwhelmed. For multimorbid, frail patients like Sonny, the intensive interventions delivered in hospital become inappropriate, and oftentimes harmful and inhumane. With sufficient capacity for care in his home, I can manage his ill-health holistically.

There is a Cinderella effect behind the demise of generalism in British medicine. What goes on in specialist services is frequently dramatic, and commands political attention. Our leaders seem obsessed with the idea that GPs can be cheaply replaced by algorithms and apps and other professionals, and that busy patients should be able to dial-a-diagnosis in much the same way as they might order a pizza. As the numbers of generalists decline, the policy has been to push nurses, pharmacists, paramedics and physicians' assistants to take their place. All are skilled and highly trained in their own roles. But none is a doctor. When someone becomes unwell, the earlier they encounter an experienced medical generalist to make a biopsychosocial diagnosis, the more appropriate and holistic their care, and the more cost-effective for the NHS as a whole. Disrupt this generalist layer in the NHS and increasing numbers of patients are sucked inappropriately into resource-intensive emergency and specialist services. This has been amply demonstrated through the gradual retreat of GPs from out-of-hours care – another New Labour folly with its origins in the 2004 GP contract – and is now being increasingly replicated in daytime general practice in many areas of the country.

This is founded on a fatal misapprehension that has prospered in the era of evidence-dictated medicine: that the diagnosis and management of illness (and risk) can be reduced to protocols and processes administrable by anyone equipped with a guideline – or even by a machine. The concept of the family doctor, so powerful when I saw my name on that set of notes on my first day as a GP principal, has barely featured in the rhetoric, reforms and redesigns that continue to emanate from the centre.

The third R is the relocation of prevention within public health. So much of what we are currently compelled to do in primary prevention – 'treating' marginally elevated blood pressures, cholesterols, HbA1cs, supported by dubious 'evidence' promulgated by vested interests – is of low or no value. Yet it consumes ever more NHS resources and workload. Alongside cholesterol, blood pressure, age and so on, one of the most important determinants of the Qrisk score (the heart disease risk calculator that so unnerved Michael in chapter 4) is your postcode. If you live in an affluent area, your risk will be lowered. If your neighbourhood is poverty-stricken, you are that much more likely to develop cardiovascular disease. This generation's challenges are the epidemic of obesity and the socioeconomic deprivation that blights so many lives. The greatest value lies in concerted measures across government to improve public health, following the model so successful in tackling tobacco. Tasking the NHS with attempting to counter the damage will fail, and will do so at a fantastic cost. Conservative governments' abhorrence of industry regulation and of legislation dismissed as 'nannying', their tolerance of spiralling food bank dependency and socioeconomic deprivation and insecurity, all have direct deleterious impacts on the NHS – to say nothing of the people affected. Their wilful ignoring of successive reports into the social determinants of health is costing all of us dear.

Re-professionalise. Rebalance. Relocate. The fourth R? The fourth R we'll come to in the final chapter. First you need to know how Marion and Ellen's stories ended.

—

Marion returned looking distinctly better. Within ten days of starting the tablets, she had noticed improvement. Now, three weeks later, her appetite was back, the nausea had gone, and the back pain and breathlessness had receded. She was relaxed, and her weight was coming back on.

Sertraline, the medication that helped her, is a potent anti-anxiety drug. We've used it on several occasions since, whenever her crippling health anxiety has flared again. With each successive episode, she has found it easier to accept the true diagnosis – anxiety – and to manage the obsessive fears about whatever terminal disease her physical symptoms so exactly represent.

Were she not to have an ongoing relationship with one doctor, her story would have been very different. On one occasion, while I was on leave, she did present to a junior colleague. Access to her notes – so-called 'informational continuity' – was no help. There is simply no possibility of reading back through more than a decade of records to try to build from scratch the picture that I carry in my head. And Marion's symptoms were every bit as alarming as they always are. An urgent referral for suspected cancer was made. Blood tests, consultant appointments, CT scans, endoscopies and biopsies all resulted. By the time Marian had finally been given the all-clear, the NHS was several thousand pounds the poorer. And she had been through the mill.

Relational continuity cannot be delivered at all times; doctors cannot be available every hour of every day. But the more it can be designed in and incentivised – the more central the place it occupies – the better served both patients and the wider NHS will be. We need sufficient numbers of doctors to deliver it. The average Norwegian GP looks after 1,200 patients and has time to properly address the challenges of multimorbidity, frailty and therapeutic complexity. The average English list size now stands at 2,200, up from around 1,800 when I entered general practice – and that was back in the era of single diseases and relative therapeutic simplicity. Primary care is currently delivered on around 8% of the total NHS budget. Pump-priming and then sustaining the redirection of just a few per cent of the existing NHS budget into general practice would recruit and retain the numbers of medical generalists needed to emulate somewhere like Norway, an investment that would repay itself several-fold in terms of reduced activity elsewhere in the system – and patient outcomes and experience would improve immeasurably.

Rebalancing generalism and specialism would also align with a central imperative: to give patients the opportunity to decide what, for them, actually has value, in terms of managing both illness and risk. Providing the information, context and support for such decisions requires time with an expert generalist, fully conversant with the bewildering complexities of the medical world and the myriad factors that interact to affect our health. Truly informed consent – with patient and clinician arriving at genuine shared decisions – returns holism to the heart of medical practice. My experience tells me that the net shift will be away from drug consumption and medicalisation towards sustainable and person-centred healthcare.

—

Ellen was delivered by Laura of a healthy baby girl, whom she and Ed named after the midwife who so generously helped her through. Literally the minute Ellen met baby Laura, she fell in love. Years' worth of fortnightly consultations with me abruptly ceased. She has blossomed with happiness again.

She still talks about Charlie, and he remains part of their family as they are going through life together. But he is the son and brother who resides in another place – distant, unreachable, but connected for all that.

I'll never know how things might otherwise have been, but having a doctor she's known for years who could allow her to express the depths of her grief and her utter ambivalence towards the new baby in her womb was certainly important. What good the super-specialised IVF and pre-implantation diagnostics were she or her child to have been crushed by the fallout from her bereavement? Our deep knowledge of her enabled midwife Laura and me to support her in a fashion that no one wielding a protocol would have countenanced, yet was exactly what Ellen needed.

13

ENDINGS

I clearly remember the words he said, and the way he said them. I was probably about fifteen. By then, my brother and sister would have been old enough to be out a lot of the time – round at friends' or attending clubs. It will have been a Tuesday. My mum taught evening classes on Tuesdays, which would have been why she wasn't there either. It was just me and Dad at home.

He came and found me. Or maybe he just came across me. I was sitting at the bottom of our stairs. It's where the phone was in our house back then, so I had probably just finished chatting to a friend. What burns bright in my mind are his words, and the tremor and the catch in his voice.

'Phil. I think the cancer's come back.'

He'd been to the loo. But instead of a normal bowel motion, there'd been a mess of bloody diarrhoea. It must have triggered flashbacks to the man dying in the bed next to him when he was recovering from his original operation. These decades later, I understand that he would have been terrified. I can see why he would have felt suddenly, awfully alone. Why he had to tell someone, whoever was around. That need will have been overwhelmingly urgent – the need to have someone connect with him, understand his fear, touch him and hold him and tell him they were sorry and that they loved him and that they were sure it was going to be all right.

But I didn't understand any of that at the time. All I saw was my father, panic-stricken. I didn't really know what cancer was. Nor did I know what it would mean if it had come back. I didn't know. I think it probably scared me, seeing him like that, though I wasn't flung into the same emotional turmoil as I was when I'd overheard him briefing Mum about their finances those years before. Maybe, in the blinkered egocentricity of adolescence, his fear repulsed me a little. I didn't touch him, nor hold him. And I certainly didn't tell him I was sorry and that I loved him. I didn't know what he needed, not back then. I didn't know what to do.

—

Discussing the ideas for this book with someone in the publishing industry – we'll call him Dan – he expressed the worry that I would simply be harking back to a bygone era, something unfitted for the modern world, something now lost which it is neither possible nor desirable to attempt to regain. His instinct was that in our busy, unboundaried lives, what matters most is swift access to advice when health concerns arise, and that antiquated notions such as continuity of care were irrelevant.

To illustrate his point, he described his experiences with a recurring bowel complaint over recent years. Evidently he was a patient at an 'industrial' practice. Every time he contacted them, he would speak to a different, unknown doctor. Who would arrange a battery of blood tests. A week later he would get a text message to tell him they were all normal. His symptoms would eventually settle, and he would carry on with life until the next time they recurred, at which point he would go through the identical loop with someone else. He seemed to think this was OK.

I could hazard a good guess at the diagnosis. And I also knew what tests each new doctor was organising, over and again – bloods to rule out coeliac disease, overactive thyroid, Crohn's and ulcerative colitis, and to make sure there was no evidence of anything potentially worrisome like anaemia. I also knew that Dan was caught in a groundhog day.

I sketched out the kind of job I would aim to do. Excluding important competing diagnoses is merely the first step. I would have followed up with him, aiming to increase his knowledge and understanding, as well as seeking to establish if he had underlying concerns as to what it all meant. I would have pointed him to reliable sources of information on the internet. We would have explored links to times of stress, and seen if there could be related dietary factors such as fermentable short-chain sugars that he might usefully cut down on or exclude.

By the time we finished the conversation, Dan had a somewhat different view of what this book might be about.

Another publishing professional – we'll call him Oliver. At the time I came to talk with him, he'd recently had an encounter with his own GP, who had advised him, following a 'health check', to go on statins. Rather than uncritically accepting the recommendation, Oliver had put his doctor on the spot, quizzing him hard as to what the actual benefits might be and what alternatives he could pursue. When I described in outline the chapters dealing with primary prevention and the medicalisation of risk, they spoke directly to his own experience. He was instantly engaged.

Re-professionalise, rebalance, relocate. The fourth R is responsibility. It is a two-sided coin. Many patients want to take responsibility for their own health. They can only do so with high-quality information, tailored to their individual context, and with a trusted guide to help them navigate what can be bewilderingly complex terrain. For that, they need clinicians with a sense of responsibility towards them, and with the opportunities, time and training to forge therapeutic relationships with them. Equally, some patients don't want, or aren't able, to assume personal responsibility. They have the same need for a doctor to be responsible – not just to take decisions on their behalf, but to do so having taken all reasonable steps to understand them as individuals, and what they value. Both government and my profession must acknowledge the erosion of responsibility that the 2004 GP contract set in train. Both must act to restore it.

I think back to myself sitting in that upstairs box room, industrial photocopier against the far wall, my Lloyd George envelope on the small square desk in front of me. Caron, the practice manager, working away in her office along the corridor. Me, reading the handwritten notes Dr Forshaw made about my perplexing illnesses as a child. Paper records are redundant and utterly unsuited to the sprawling, hugely complex world of modern medicine. Computerisation and technology have brought untold benefits and will further do so. But to me, those buff-coloured folders are emblematic of something that remains as important today as it was back then, even though both doctors and patients have become very different things. They speak of the doctor–patient relationship at the heart of medicine, the humanity of what healthcare should involve. It is something we have been losing over the decades of my career, but which it is both possible and imperative to regain.

—

Dad was wrong. There was a flurry of appointments with the gastroenterologists, but the bloody diarrhoea that he'd feared meant his cancer had returned proved to be something else entirely, an inflammatory condition of the bowel. His doctors treated him for ulcerative colitis, though the cause was probably the radiotherapy that had earlier helped to save his life. Radiotherapy was still relatively unsophisticated in the late 1960s, and high doses across a wide field may have caused injury to his bowel that manifested itself as a late colitis.

He survived to see his children grow up and become a computer programmer, a teacher and a doctor. Grandchildren were born. He kept working as a civil servant for a number of years, but the combined toll of his physical and psychological traumas eventually led to early retirement. Freed from the stresses of commuting and work, he went on to enjoy perhaps the best period of health he had known for decades. Even the colitis, amazingly, resolved.

I was a partner in my Oxford practice by the time new difficulties arose. He was sixty-eight. The skin over the bottom of his back – in the area of his old radiotherapy field – started to break down and refused to heal despite a plastic surgeon's best efforts at grafting. Then a blood test by his

GP picked up a problem with his liver. An ultrasound scan found extensive metastases. A biopsy revealed an aggressive, poorly differentiated cancer that might have arisen originally from squamous skin cells.

It's a long-recognised problem with radiotherapy: thirty to thirty-five years after treatment, the radiation that once saved life causes a new cancer to form.

—

Continuity with a good general practitioner is vital if we want to experience holistic care. A system, a protocol, a guideline – they are by definition impersonal. The GP, steeped in the medical world, intimately acquainted with the ways in which the NHS works and sometimes lets us down, and equally conversant with the myriad interplay between biology and emotions, psychology and life circumstances in the experience of illness – the GP is our expert ally.

This book is not about self-preservation, not in a professional sense. I will play out the last decade of my career, continuing to try to answer in relation to my patients: what should a doctor be? My daughter Pippa is at the other end of her life in medicine and she will find her own path. Like all talented and capable entrants of her generation she has options. She may well decide to follow a hospital career: she's interested in anaesthetics and critical care. If the NHS proves not to be a sustainable system in which to work, she might decide to move abroad. Or, if the way she's expected to practise medicine precludes the person-centred care she is motivated by, she may switch to another profession entirely.

This book is written for patients, of which I – all of us – are one. My mother is now in her mid-eighties and progressively frail with a number of health conditions. I am thankful that her own GP provides the kind of continuity and person-centred care that serves her well. He has protected her from pointless medicalisation and investigation on any number of occasions, while attending to the things that are of value to her. She has implicit trust and faith in him, and with my medical hat on I see that time and again his judgements have been spot on. I also know how endangered a species he has become.

I am fortunate still to enjoy good health but illness will inevitably come – as it will for you and for your loved ones. When it does, we should all expect to have a doctor like that to rely on.

—

Dad saw an oncologist with the result of the liver biopsy, who said he could give him some generic chemotherapy which had about a 20% chance of buying him a few more months, albeit that any extra time gained would be marred by the side effects of treatment. He discussed it with Mum, and with his GP, and after weighing the pros and cons, he decided it wasn't worth it. He returned home and prepared to die.

I was no longer that ignorant fifteen-year-old boy. I told him I loved him more than once and touched on the things about him that I admired – what a great job he'd done as a dad to us in spite of everything he'd been through. Our relationship had never been entirely easy, the health problems he'd endured had made it so. And in the end I didn't get to say goodbye in the way I would ideally have liked. But at least I knew roughly what to do.

We gathered the family for one last Christmas, all his grandchildren too. He was still in reasonably good shape – it would be some months before the cancer overwhelmed. Memories were made, memories were shared. I knew he dreaded what was to come, that he was haunted by his memories of that wasted man dying in the bed next to his, those thirty-five years before.

We were all still down there shortly after New Year. I went from our rented holiday cottage to be with him when his trusted GP came round for a review, along with the Macmillan nurse from the local hospice. After they'd gone, he wanted to sleep – he'd had very little the night before. Mum and I stayed talking in the sitting room for a while, then I decided it was time to head back to rejoin my brood.

I'd left my coat on the hook on the back of his bedroom door, so I crept in quietly so as not to disturb him. I glanced across to see if he was stirring and instantly recognised that he had gone. A heart attack, probably, while he was fast asleep; he wouldn't have known a thing. He had been spared the drawn-out death he had so long dreaded. And I was on hand to break the news and to support my mum.

A NOTE ON THE TEXT

I have focused on a few specific conditions, principally ischaemic heart disease, heart failure, and type 2 diabetes, to illustrate the transformations that have occurred in medicine since my journey as a doctor began. Comparable revolutions have occurred in virtually every area of practice.

Where I have described the origins of atherosclerosis (the 'furring up' of arteries) I have uncritically drawn on the 'cholesterol hypothesis' which currently dominates medical thinking and practice, and which has become embedded in popular understanding of the causation of heart disease. It is however almost certainly wrong. It was beyond the scope of this book to examine the debate, but interested readers should seek out the work of Dr Malcolm Kendrick, particularly *The Great Cholesterol Con* and *The Clot Thickens*, which offer alternative perspectives on this fascinating area.

All the patient stories in this book are 'true', but have been anonymised and fictionalised to protect identity. In many cases, characters are composites. The scenarios presented will be familiar to every GP in the land.

Where I have interviewed fellow professionals their identity is real, except for the few instances where there was concern over potential impacts on career. Where anonymisation has occurred, I have indicated this in the text. The GP registrars who feature in several stories have all been given pseudonyms.

I am grateful to Jason Maude and his daughter Isabel, who kindly allowed me to relate their family's story in chapter 6.

My own family's story is also presented without anonymisation, and I am grateful to my mum, sister, brother and my daughters for their support in the creation of this book. *What Is a Doctor?* is something I am certain my dad would have been wholeheartedly behind as well.

ACKNOWLEDGEMENTS

Many people have influenced and contributed to this book. First and foremost are my patients, who continue to teach me valuable lessons on a daily basis. I am constantly mindful that it is my privilege to serve them as their doctor.

I owe a huge debt of thanks to Jason Cowley, editor-in-chief of the *New Statesman*, without whom *What Is a Doctor?* would not exist. Jason has given me the opportunity to develop my thinking and writing about medicine in the pages of the *New Statesman* over the past decade. He strongly encouraged me to write this book and provided pivotal feedback during the early stages of its development.

I am very grateful to all the colleagues who agreed to be interviewed. Two deserve special mention. Denis Pereira Gray has given generously of his time and wisdom, and his indefatigable advocacy for the proper practice of medicine has been a source of inspiration. Peter Tate, my trainer when I was a fledgling GP in the mid-1990s, has easily been the most influential figure in my professional life. If I have any useful insights on the predicament of medicine today, their origins can be traced to Peter and what he taught me both as his registrar and subsequently over our correspondence and conversations.

Huge thanks, too, to Dr Simon Crouch – my brother-in-law and an eminent medical statistician at the University of York – who provided much apposite criticism. I have failed to do justice to (among others) his comprehensive analysis of the ways in which corporate, academic and political interests corrupt and compromise the production, interpretation and implementation of scientific 'evidence', to say nothing of the parlous state of public health in this country. In mitigation, these areas are, as Simon points out, worthy of books all of their own.

Andrew Gordon at David Higham Associates saw potential in this book at an early stage, and provided exceptional help in developing the project and seeing it through to publication. I'm grateful to Helen Bleck for her meticulous copyediting, and for ironing out numerous infelicities in my prose. In Simon Thorogood and the entire team at Canongate I have been 'a fortunate man' indeed. They brought enthusiasm and belief to the project from the get-go, and Simon has provided invaluable editorial input to develop it into the book it is today.